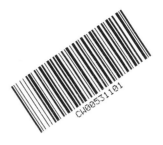

THE COFFEE CURE DIET

Live Longer and Look Younger

by

Justus Robert Hope, M.D.

Featuring the

Lacto-Mediterranean Lifestyle

Published by Hope Pressworks International, LLC, Redding, California.

Printed in the United States of America. No part of this book may be used or reproduced in any manner whatsoever, whether electronic or mechanical or stored in a database or retrieval system, without written permission except in the case of brief quotations embodied in critical articles and reviews. For information, address Hope Pressworks International LLC, P.O. Box 991216, Redding, California, 96099-1216.

First Edition

Library of Congress Cataloging-in-Publication Data has been applied for.

ISBN: 978-0-9980554-5-9

The information presented in this book is the result of years of practice, experience, and clinical research by the author. However, it is not a substitute for evaluation and treatment by a medical doctor. The information contained herein is for educational purposes only. It is not intended to be a substitute for professional medical advice. The reader should always consult with his or her physician to determine the appropriateness of the information for his or her own medical situation and treatment plan. Reading this book does not constitute a physician-patient relationship. The stories in this book are true. The names and circumstances of the stories have been changed at times to preserve privacy.

Cover Design by Daniel Ojedokun

CONTENTS

DEDICATION

This book would not have been possible without two people, Dr. Gerald Reaven, the scientist who discovered the condition of insulin resistance, and my wife, Faith, who introduced me to the Adventist diet. Dr. Reaven introduced the world to the metabolic syndrome, originally known as syndrome X in 1988, a condition from which I suffered. Now, approximately half of the population of the United States is similarly afflicted, as well as another one billion people worldwide. The Coffee Cure Diet is not just an effective tool for weight loss; it is a formidable weapon against insulin resistance. For most, it will be helpful, but for many, like me, it will be life-saving.

Justus R. Hope, M.D.
Redding, California
July 2019

INTRODUCTION

Just before my 60th birthday and my 32 years of medical practice, it was time to write this book; a book on diet and exercise, and more importantly, as my research directed me, a book on coffee.

Before I decided upon a career in medicine, while still a teenager, I was already obsessed with health and the analysis of why some people lived longer than others. After studying medicine at Baylor College of Medicine in Houston and completing a residency at the University of California, Irvine, I read everything that I could get my hands on concerning heart disease and cancer prevention.

Over the years some scientific advice on health has remained the same. For example: vegetarian diets are healthier than meat-based ones, those who exercise live longer, and cigarette smoking shortens life. Over the past 40 years the science has also flip-flopped on other recommendations. For example: alcohol, once thought to be unhealthy, can actually decrease heart attack risk if used in moderation. Conversely, aerobic exercise, once thought to be universally healthy, can cause oxidative stress and inflammation. Most interestingly, coffee drinking, far from being an addictive and unhealthy habit, has now been shown to lower the risk of death from all causes. In short, coffee drinking can help people live longer.

To be sure, there are still a fair amount of skeptics about the benefits of coffee, even among physicians. But my own personal story, though anecdotal, shows exactly how coffee can improve one's health. At age 42, I struggled with health and weight control. My blood pressure was out of control despite medications. No matter what diet I tried, I was always 25-30 pounds overweight. The first place I gained was my waist, and it was the last place that I lost. I had tried vegetarianism, keto, low carb, Atkins, low-fat, and calorie counting. Nothing worked.

So I started going to the gym five days a week. I jogged and even tried weight lifting. I ate healthy (or so I thought). No red meat, just chicken and fish. I drank no coffee or wine at that time, because I did not want to worsen my blood pressure or increase my risk for heart attack. Despite all of this, my health continued to worsen. I became pre-diabetic. I got out of breath easily. My memory grew foggy. At age 42, despite medication, exercise, and a so-called healthy diet, my body fat hovered close to 30%. My blood pressure was 160/100. My waist ballooned to 38 inches, and my cholesterol rose to 200.

Today, at age 62, my body fat is closer to 15%. My weight is 20 pounds less, and my waist is 34 inches. My blood pressure is down to 99/69, and my cholesterol is barely 97. I am the happiest I have ever been, and my health is better than when I was 20. I spend 80% less time today exercising, and I drink wine. Coffee, however, proved to be the secret to my success.

In the pages that follow, allow me to share with you the most important discovery that I have made in my career.

Two Ways to Read This Book

Much of this book is written at the scientific level, to explain concepts such as oxidation and inflammation, to explain differences in the genetics of obesity, and to reflect the mountain of scientific evidence supporting the Coffee Cure components. For those who are not interested in this, simply focus on the basic chapters like Chapter 3: The Coffee Cure Diet Plan and Chapter 8: Coffee Cure Tips & Tactics. Or simply read Section I.

For the regular guy patient who simply wants to do the program, focus on Phases I and II in Chapter 3, and with your doctor's approval, begin the four pillars of the program. Pillars 1 and 2 require drinking a mixture of coffee and whey protein before each meal. Pillar 3 involves timed meals known as time-restricted eating, essentially consuming all one's meals in an eight-hour window. Pillar 4 involves resistive exercises like pulling on stretch bands. This involves a time commitment of about 15 to 25 minutes per day.

For those who cannot do all the pillars; even three out of four will produce weight loss and an improvement in health. For example, those who cannot tolerate coffee can still drink whey protein shakes before each meal with good benefit. The four-pillar approach is designed to lower appetite, lower inflammation, reduce oxidation, and post-meal blood fat and blood sugar surges. It is targeted to reduce insulin resistance, visceral fat, and the risk for diabetes.

The Coffee Cure Diet program is designed to be an easy intervention for those individuals wishing to shed the unhealthy Western diet and lifestyle. All diets can be rated in four categories:

#1. Effectiveness of weight loss
#2. Ease of use
#3. Effect on health
#4. Risk of weight regain

Some diets produce rapid weight loss, such as the low carb, the fasting approach, diet pills, or bariatric surgery (if you can call that a diet). Ten pounds or more a month is considered rapid. The Coffee Cure often produces rapid weight loss, but that is not the end goal.

Ease of use is the second category. An example of a difficult diet would be trying to suddenly switch to vegan after years of eating meat. This would be difficult to impossible for most. Calorie cutting can be difficult; for example trying to cut 500 calories per day was very tough for me. I hated being hungry. Taking diet pills, by comparison, was very easy.

Drinking your diet pill in the form of the Coffee Cure is just as easy. Qualifying for bariatric surgery and undergoing an operation is very difficult—definitely not easy. I felt the low-carb meat diet was easy as well. The only problem was that it was not all that healthy. In fact, high-fat diets can produce insulin resistance and are associated with a higher rate of diabetes and cancer.

Speaking as both a human being and a physician, this third category, health, was of the utmost importance to me. That is why I devote at least half of this book to the Coffee Cure's effect on your health, your body on the Coffee Cure. I break it down to the Coffee Cure's effects on various organ systems. The Coffee Cure is right up there as one of the healthiest weight-loss approaches, next to the Mediterranean diet and the vegetarian approach.

The final category, number 4, is the chance of relapse; that is, regaining all the weight lost, and often more. This is where most diets fail. Some fail more miserably than others. Pure fasting diets fail because at some point the fast ends and there is a rapid regain of water, electrolytes, and fat. When a diet ends, usually the body compensates for the lowered weight with increased hunger and reduced metabolism which predictably results in weight regain.

Diets that combine exercise with weight loss suffer less in this category. The Coffee Cure has built in relapse-prevention strategies with the focus on increasing metabolism and suppressing appetite. As you read the program, keep in mind that the Coffee Cure is the only diet I know that scores high in all four categories; that is, effectiveness, ease of use, benefit to health, and low risk of relapse.

SECTION I:

THE COFFEE CURE

Chapter 1

THE METABOLIC SYNDROME

"I feel better and have more energy." -Byron T.

"Eggs and bacon," Byron told me matter-of-factly. "Everyday at noon. That's it, doc."

"Anything else?" I asked.

"Nope."

"No bread or salad?"

"Nothing."

"So, let me get this straight, Byron. You eat once every 24 hours, and all you eat are eggs and bacon?"

"Yeah. And I can't seem to lose anymore weight."

"How much have you lost?" I asked.

"Well, I am down almost 40 pounds since my heart surgery, but I am at a plateau now. I tried fasting for a whole week and lost 14 pounds. Then, as soon as I started eating, it all came back in a few days."

"Have you tried a couple of smaller meals instead of one large one meal per day?"

"Yeah, I ate six small meals in eight hours, and gained 12 pounds, so I went back to once a day. Last week my girlfriend talked me into having a Cobb salad, and the next day I was up seven pounds."

***

Byron was a patient of mine who suffered from the metabolic syndrome, where one gains all their weight in the middle. Those with metabolic syndrome form visceral (or abdominal) fat, the most dangerous kind of fat, and they tend to develop heart attacks, strokes, cancers, and dementia.

Byron had been lucky. His life was saved with a four-vessel coronary bypass surgery. Following the procedure, the doctors told him he needed to stop eating the fatty, greasy fast foods. Afraid for his life, he did—for about five years. Slowly he relapsed into his old familiar and satisfying habits: burgers, fries, steaks, hash browns, and pork sausage.

He went back to his job as a car mechanic, and he did well until the weight and chest pain returned. Speaking as a pain specialist, I didn't normally see heart patients, but I agreed to see Byron when he developed chest pain from the incision made during the bypass surgery.

Byron didn't much trust doctors, and I really couldn't blame him. Most doctors are not pictures of health themselves, nor do they provide sound nutritional advice. Most weight-loss doctors I knew pushed diet pills, which can lead to heart problems. Bariatric surgery, or surgically shrinking the stomach to the size of a walnut, is now all the modern medical rage. One of my patients once referred it to a forced diet, because if you try to overeat—even once—you are severely punished by stabbing pains. The weight loss occurs very fast following the surgery, often leading to sagging and wrinkled skin. Many patients develop osteoporosis and fractures. In other cases, the weight inexorably returns as the patient learns to drink their calories in walnut-sized servings.

In my own journey to get healthy, I also was disappointed by the traditional medical advice, despite being a physician. Over the years the medical profession has advocated one weight-loss approach after another, ranging from restricting calories to avoiding processed foods, to engaging in regular physical activity. Virtually all of them have failed the average patient and resulted in increasing numbers with diabetes and the dreaded metabolic syndrome. These numbers used to include me, but now they included Byron.

Because Byron was leery of doctors, he tended to miss appointments and stop medications. He didn't care for pills or prescriptions. He put most of his faith in Google. He believed in Paleo, Keto, and grass-fed beef. He was a do-it-yourselfer through and through. No matter what he did, he just couldn't keep the weight off.

Where did Byron go wrong? Here was a man in his late 50s with a heart attack, a four-way bypass, and high blood pressure trying to stay alive. He was single and didn't like to cook, so he ate fast food. He had read about how fats were "good" for you, but he didn't differentiate between saturated and unsaturated fats. Saturated fats are different than "good" plant fats as they are not liquid at room temperature. Bacon fat or the grease from cooking a steak hardens to a Crisco-like substance at room temperature. Studies have shown that saturated fats are toxic and pro-inflammatory, associated with not only heart disease but also many other diseases including dementia and cancers. They are terrible for your health.

In addition to his one-meal-a-day fasting, Byron was sold on the Keto diet, one that derives most of its calories from proteins and fats. There are some potential health benefits from this approach, but the problem is that it is high in fats—and, in Byron's case, saturated fats. Because fruits and vegetables contain carbohydrates, many keto patients eat little or none of these foods, leading to further diseases and deficiencies.

Byron did not realize that prolonged fasting and ketosis can lead to muscle loss. In the short term, as most keto books point out, this does not occur. Speaking from my own deep personal experience, I can tell you that my arm and leg muscles shriveled down as I practiced the keto diet for some five years. In someone like Byron or my former self, high insulin levels are the common denominator of the condition. The high insulin levels prevent the belly or visceral fat from being burned, so it accumulates. In ketosis the body prefers to break down muscle, leading to the appearance that we typically see in metabolic syndrome, which now affects 35% of the United States population and a growing percentage of the world's population. Arms and legs wither as the waist thickens.

As if this weren't bad enough, Byron's metabolism had slowed to the pace of a snail. Most people, some 80%, quickly regain the weight lost after a diet. Look no further than the fate of the contestants on NBC's *The Biggest Loser*. 80% regained their weight within one year of the show. Why did the 20% keep their weight off? The simple answer is "metabolism." The good news is that you can change your metabolism like they did.

There are a few ways to increase a sluggish metabolism. The easiest way is one that does not require exercise and involves simply consuming more protein. I would not advise eating protein combined with saturated fat, like beef or steak. Instead, I recommend whey protein.

The studies on whey protein are also clear. It is healthy, and it is associated with a host of health benefits like anti-oxidation and anti-inflammation. It helps with the processing and metabolism of carbohydrates. Most importantly it creates a thermic effect.

Fat produces no significant thermic effect. If one consumes 100 calories of fat, the body gains access to 97 of those calories. Only 3 calories are required to metabolize the fat. For carbohydrates the story is similar with about 10 calories being required to burn them. For every 100 calories of protein consumed, however, fully 30 calories are expended to utilize it, causing an increase in metabolism and assisting with weight maintenance.

I recommended that Byron supplement his diet with 40-60 grams of whey protein per day. This is NOT a high protein diet. Assuming a 2,000 calorie per day intake, the supplement represents little more than a 10% protein diet. Whey and casein are the two proteins which comprise milk. Casein is the solid portion or curd, while the liquid portion is the whey.

In a study of 100 individuals who lost 30 pounds, one-half were given a regular carbohydrate energy drink while the other one-half were given 45 grams of a whey-protein supplement. At the end of six months, the carbohydrate group had regained seven pounds (almost all of it fat), while the whey group regained only one and a half pounds (all of it muscle).[1]

When even a little exercise is added, weight maintenance becomes even easier. A study showed that just 30 minutes of resistive training, or RT, raised resting metabolism not only for a few hours after exercise, but for more than 24 hours. Thirty minutes of RT raised basal metabolism by 10-12% even 24 hours later.[2]

During weight maintenance, I strongly advise a workout of 20 sets of 20 repetitions like the one I developed for Byron. It is designed to get blood to flow through the muscles and raise one's metabolism. It is simple, easy, and can be incorporated into your daily routine and accomplished in your home.

The Coffee Cure

The other problem with Byron's diet was eating only once per day; this signaled his body that he was in "calorie conservation mode," otherwise known as starvation. His body's metabolism slowed to burn as little energy as possible while his system attempted to store as much fat as possible. By eating even a little food over three meals spread over eight hours, one signals the body that food is once again plentiful, and the body can return to "normal mode." This is where metabolism is restored and fat is no longer hoarded.

It is here that the coffee's miraculous properties come into play. In addition to all the other health benefits that studies have shown, coffee is also an effective appetite suppressant. Drinking a cup of coffee before each meal will help you eat less even as you eat more frequently, keeping your body's metabolism in "normal mode" as long as possible.

I changed Byron's diet to three meals, the first involving an egg, coffee, and a whey protein-based creamer. The second would be two hours later, involving an apple with coffee and whey protein. The third, which was dinner, was still his usual two eggs and bacon, but this time it was turkey bacon and came with a cup of coffee and whey protein.

I also placed Byron on a circuit exercise program for 30 minutes each day focusing on arms, legs, and chest using bands and light dumb bells (5-10 pounds). Such muscle strengthening exercise will also revive a sluggish metabolism. I find it does so more easily and effectively than aerobic exercise or plain walking.

Finally, I advised Byron to change his fasting style to 16-hour fasts, four days per week. These fasts do not slow metabolism like longer ones. Such daily fasts are a form of intermittent fasting, known as TRE or Time-Restricted Eating. TRE is a form of daily fasting where one restricts all of their meals and calories to an eight-hour window. From the last bite of food one day to the first bite of food the next day; a full 16 hours should elapse. The studies on TRE for five days per week are clear. A 2018 study looked at 18 hour time-restricted eating in a group of men with prediabetes, similar to Byron. They were compared to themselves. First they ate in a 12 hour window for five weeks. Later they crossed over to an 18-hour time-restricted eating schedule for five weeks. TRE improved blood pressure, insulin sensitivity, and oxidative stress, all of which are heavily associated with cardiovascular disease.[3]

I sent Byron home with this prescription, and I told him to come back in a few weeks. As it turned out, the four pillars of the Coffee Cure—coffee, time-restricted eating, whey protein and RT supplementation—were precisely what he needed.

When Byron came to see me three weeks later, I asked him how it was going.

"I feel better." he said. "I was down over fifteen pounds after a couple of weeks. I can't believe it doc; when I got down to 156, I had to weigh myself three times to make sure the scale was working. I thought it was broken. You know, I have been wanting to wear my size 29 jeans for years, but even with the 40 pound weight loss before I started with you, I couldn't. When I saw the scales at 156, I figured I would try them on, and you know what, they fit."

"How did that make you feel, Byron?" I couldn't believe it. You broke your plateau. Congratulations!

Then he looked at me and said, "And for some reason when I look at things, they seem brighter and clearer."

"I know," I said.

Chapter 2

THRIFTY GENES, SKINNY GENES

"My blood pressure has lowered with this program." —Bill J.

Byron and I are like millions of other Americans; problems with weight are simply in our genes. But not everyone is like us. Before you embark on your Coffee Cure journey, it's important to understand how your body is genetically programmed to respond to changes in diet.

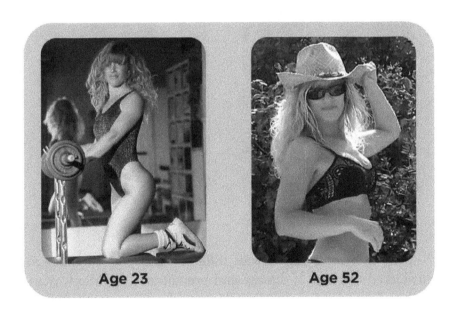

Age 23   Age 52

My wife, Faith, looks as slim as her brother (the doctor) and her mother (the grandma). All three have less than 15% body fat, eat anything they want, and never gain an ounce. They also are human dynamos; preferring to never rest. Watching them can make one dizzy. All three look younger than their age, and they clearly have a low risk of disease. Is it something in their genes?

When we first met, it was Faith's jeans that attracted me. But after I noticed her Levi's, I was stunned by her tiny waist. Faith had a waist to hip ratio of less than 0.7 and closer to 0.65. This was certainly attractive to look at, but it was also a powerful indicator of health. Those with IR tend to gain visceral fat, where this key ratio is a little higher. Men with metabolic syndrome have ratios closer to 0.9, while women with the disease have ratios greater than 0.85.

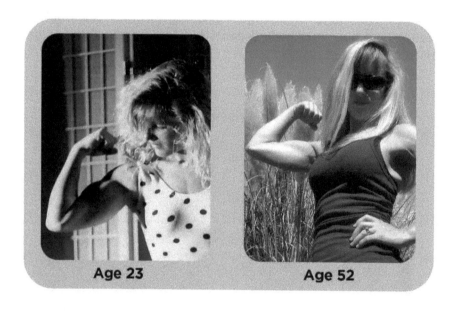

Age 23   Age 52

Belly fat is correlated with inflammation and IR. Both are considered markers of disease and premature aging. So why was Faith so lucky and I so unlucky? Because she did an excellent job of choosing her parents.

Most people who suffer from the metabolic syndrome have to overcome their genetic tendencies. Faith did not have to try. At age 54 she still wears size 0 and trades clothes with her 21-year-old daughter.

My patients invariably ask Faith, "What do you eat to look like that?"

She answers, "Chips and dip and lots of cheese and beans."

"You must be starving to stay so thin," they say.

She answers, "No, I eat what I want."

Granted, Faith and her entire family are Seventh-Day Adventists, and they subscribe to a lacto-ovo-vegetarian diet – one of the healthiest diets on the planet. She has drunk coffee for years, and without realizing it consumed whey protein through her intake of dairy such as cheese. She tends to avoid breakfast, so her first food intake is almost always more than 16 hours after her last bite the previous day. She hates sweets except for dark chocolates. She prefers body-building to endurance training. In other words, without purposefully doing it, Faith has been on the Coffee Cure Diet her entire life. Anyone can do this program.

Faith: Coffee Cure Ground Zero

Admittedly, I was not a vegetarian when I met Faith, but peer pressure has a way of motivating you. At first, I enjoyed steak fajitas once a week, and I also enjoyed a box of chocolate covered peanuts. Let's just say that now I have been off all meat for around three years and have not eaten a single chocolate covered peanut.

Don't get me wrong, I occasionally have pizza or chicken wings or turkey burger once a month for family outings or barbeques, but I don't eat beef and I don't eat sweets anymore. Not because I fight a craving. No, it is because I enjoy the bean dip more. It is because I have lost my belly fat.

The longer you go without sugar, the less you crave it, and the same is true for meat. Now whenever I indulge in my barbeque chicken wings once a month, I have to restrict my portion to two pieces or I will feel ill. Once you develop healthy habits, your appetite normalizes.

I used to feel tired and sluggish and wanted to veg-out all day Saturday watching television. Now I drink coffee and try to keep up with Faith's gardening. I chop firewood, clean the pool, mow the lawn, etc. Just because I wasn't born with great genes doesn't mean that I can't look like and act like I was. One can reduce the expression of bad genes with environment, like coffee drinking, diet changes, and more physical activity.

I simply have turned my bad genes off and activated my good genes. I don't just look like I did. My numbers and health prove it. My dentist of 20 years recently asked why my gums suddenly were no longer inflamed, and the pockets had actually regressed. "This never happens," he said. My patients who adopt the Coffee Cure also notice similar reductions in inflammation; even my lean patients who take it up require less pain medication to treat conditions like inflammatory arthritis.

Activate Your Good Genes

Fake it until you make it someone once said, but why do I have to try when those who were born lucky like my wife, Faith, never seem to? George Burns could eat anything and stay thin. He could even smoke and drink and never have to pay the price. He lived to be 100.

The answer once again is related to our two primary drivers of disease; inflammation and oxidation. Those of us born with excellent genetics can eat anything and never gain an ounce, while the majority of us with mediocre or negative genes cannot. Studies of identical twins have shown that even those born with fat genes can be thin if they are purposeful with their diet and exercise.

What exactly is the main difference in genetics, you might ask? What are the key features that separate good from bad genes, or for that matter, fat from skinny genes? Great question, and to the best of my research and knowledge there are two answers.

The first is the theory that the world evolved into two populations. Those like me who would succeed in times of famine, who could eat very little and yet still not lose precious weight, and those who would succeed in times of food abundance, like Faith.

The thrifty gene groups, like Byron and me, conserve energy by always preferring to rest, take naps, lay on the couch and eat. They pack on weight easily and store it effortlessly. If they were saving money instead of energy, they would be wealthy. But in times of plenty, like in our current Western culture, they succumb to diseases such as type II diabetes, metabolic syndrome, related cancers, and cardiovascular diseases.

By contrast, those with skinny genes, like Faith and her brother and like George Burns, prefer to stay active almost to the point of hyperactivity. They are in perpetual motion either at their jobs or at their leisure. When they are not hiking, cycling, running, surfing, or training, they are puttering around the home, trimming hedges, stacking boxes, and planting a garden. They seldom have time for eating, and they are always thin.

In famines, this group of people might starve because they spend their energy freely while not saving. In times of abundance, like our modern Western culture, those with the skinny genes tend to outlive those of us with thrifty genes. Most of us readily identify with one of these two main types.

THRIFY GENES' TRAITS

- Very good at saving calories; holds on to them
- Prefers sitting on couch over walk in park
- Enjoys fatty or sugary foods
- Often returns for second portion
- Cleans plate

SKINNY GENES' TRAITS

- Poor at saving calories; wastes them freely
- Prefers walk in park over sitting on couch
- Often forgets to eat. Low interest in food
- Often leaves food on plate
- Never eats seconds

The second reason that those with skinny genes are different from us is that they have low levels of inflammation and oxidation. It is not necessarily because they live a healthier lifestyle. Take George Burns for example; he smoked his entire life and this habit usually creates massive inflammation and oxidation (oxidized LDL particles). But not in George. Those with skinny genes tend to have very low levels of LDL and high levels of the protective HDL. Whenever George ate and fats and sugars surged in his bloodstream, those levels were quickly neutralized.

THRIFY GENES' HEALTH

- Often obese or overweight
- Elevated inflammation
- High rates of metabolic disease
- Often premature death

SKINNY GENES' HEALTH

- Lean or normal weight
- Low levels of inflammation
- Low rates of disease
- Often long lived

George Burns did not have any belly fat. Neither does Faith. Her waist circumference, the last time I measured it, was a scant 23 inches, even at age 54.

How do you approach life if you are like me, born with high triglycerides or a thick waist? As I said earlier, you fake it until you make it. You do everything in your power to look and act like a person with skinny genes. You make sure that your weight stays in the normal range. You burn calories by mimicking the habits of a naturally thin person. In short, you try to prevent the fat genes from expressing themselves by refusing to provide them with ammunition, the extra calories.

FAKE IT UNTIL YOU MAKE IT

- Imitate the habits of a skinny-genes person
- Use coffee and whey to curb appetite and cravings
- Use coffee to energize and stay off couch
- Use coffee/whey to extend the time between meals

I take my cues from Faith. If she doesn't want a second bowl of soup, I try to avoid a second bowl as well. If I have trouble fighting the urge, I simply drink another cup of coffee with some whey protein. If I am still hungry I make a bargain with myself. I allow myself one-half of an extra serving. If I am still hungry after that, I add a quarter of an extra serving.

If Faith wants to trim hedges, yet I feel like lying on the couch, the same thing. I have a strong cup of coffee – without whey – as I am going for energy not appetite suppression. The java jolt energizes me, and I go outside and get physical. If the television is still calling my name an hour later, then I bargain with myself. I'll watch a one-hour show, and then go back outside for a swim in the pool.

***

As a person with bad genes, I am perpetually haunted by the legendary story of Jeanne Calment and André-Francois Raffray. In 1965, Mr. Raffray, an attorney, decided to strike a deal to purchase a grand apartment near Marseilles in the South of France. Not having a lot of money, he was able to get a "deal" by purchasing the apartment on the "Enviager" or "for life" for the sum of 2,500 francs (about $500 per month). Mr. Raffray would be entitled to receive ownership of the apartment upon the seller's death. Since Jeanne Calment was age 90 at the time of the deal and Raffray only 47, it seemed like Mr. Raffray would have a steal worthy of any attorney's praise. But alas, 15 years passed and Mr. Raffray aged from 47 to 62, and the work of the law took its toll on his not so perfect genetics. Meanwhile, Jeanne Calment, a cigarette smoker, continued to defy the odds and was alive and well at age 105. She enjoyed her apartment and the $90,000 of spending money courtesy of the generous attorney Raffray.

Another fifteen years passed by and the year was 1995. Another $90,000 richer, Jeanne Calment was still alive. This was no doubt because she had chosen to give up smoking for "health reasons" following her hip fracture. Mr. Raffray bought the farm in 1995 at the ripe old age of 77. At the time of his death, Raffray had paid $184,000 to Jeanne Calment, twice the value of the apartment, and her genetics had gotten the best of the poor lawyer. Raffray's heirs continued to pay Jeanne until she passed two years later at the respectable age of 122 ½ years.

Know Your Levels

Mr. Raffray was confident that he would outlive Jeanne Calment, yet was oblivious to the fact that his genetics were not as sturdy as hers. Today, we have excellent medical science that can tell us where we stand. One should always be aware of one's crucial numbers. Know your killer micron levels like total cholesterol, LDL, HDL, and triglycerides.

If you have a ratio of total cholesterol to HDL three or less, you will probably live a long time as this reflects low levels of inflammation and oxidation provided that you do not mess it up by smoking or doing drugs.

At age 32, my numbers were terrible. My ratio of total cholesterol to HDL was eight. 200 for cholesterol and 25 for HDL. Today at age 61, my ratio is down to 2.25. Total cholesterol 95 and HDL 42.

You will also want another key ratio, your TG/HDL ratio, as low as possible, preferably under 3.0.

Studies show substantially greater atherosclerotic plaque formation when the ratio of TG/HDL is greater than 3.5. Researchers bred mice to have the Apo protein E gene negative causing a four–fold increase in their triglycerides. Despite these terrible genetics, whey protein supplementation dramatically lowered the TG levels while increasing the HDL levels of the mice. The whey-supplemented Apo-E mice had 31% less atherosclerotic plaque formation.[4]

The lesson here is in spite of the worst genetics, whey and coffee can help level the playing field for survival.

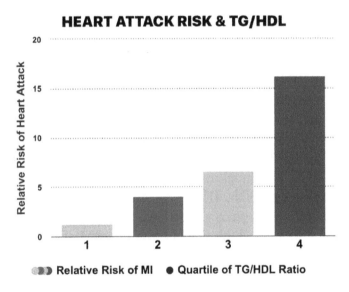

Adapted from Guizano et al. Circulation. 1997.

Figure 1. The Triglyceride/HDL Ratio

Know your blood pressure and fasting glucose. If your pressure is less than 110/70, then congratulations. If your fasting blood sugar is less than 90 and your triglycerides are below 100, then double congratulations. You are in the minority with excellent genetics.

On the other hand, if your pressure is greater than 130/85 or your blood sugar is above 100, or your triglycerides are above 150, you may have the same bad genes I was born with.

My favorite ratio is the Triglyceride divided by HDL Ratio. I refer to it as "The Longevity Index" as I will soon explain. You will need two numbers from one blood test. The first number is your HDL. This tells us how much of the "good cholesterol" you have. Your HDL acts as a scavenger to bind to killer microns and through reverse-cholesterol transport get rid of them.

The second number is your serum triglyceride. This tells us how much blood fat you have. Those with thrifty genes often have high numbers for triglycerides and low numbers for HDL. The most important single number is the ratio of TG/HDL. Ratios higher than 3 are associated with dementia and premature death from heart disease. I like to glance at an HDL number and predict how long someone will live. Many people make it to their age in their HDL serum level.

My Swiss step-grandfather made it to age 105, and he had the highest male HDL I had ever seen, a level of 92. His triglycerides were low, very healthy, at 65. His ratio was 65/92 or 0.70, one of the best I had seen. No wonder he lived so long.

My other patient Dale, whose story is told later, had horrible numbers, similar to mine. He had an HDL of 35, meaning I would not have given him much more than 35 years until he developed severe disease or death. His triglycerides were elevated at 245, making his ratio 245/35 or 7. Anything over 3 is unhealthy, but 7 is associated with a very high risk of heart attack. Dale died at age 58 after multiple amputations and severe diabetic complications.

My triglycerides were 250 at age 30 with an HDL of 25. That gave me a ratio of 250/25 or 10. Much worse than Dale's. I did not realize it at the time, nor did my doctor because insulin resistance had not yet been discovered. By those numbers, I would have given myself odds of almost a certain heart attack at an early age, maybe not 25, but for sure before age 50. Studies show that those with my ratio of TG/HDL had risks of atherosclerosis five-fold higher than those with low ratios.

I was lucky and changed my diet, my health, and my habits. Now my triglycerides are down to 120 and my HDL is up to 42. My ratio is now a respectable 120/42 or 2.9. I may make it a few more years, but only because of the Coffee Cure.

As for Faith, I would have expected numbers reflecting excellent genetics and health. And she surpassed those expectations. Her triglycerides are only 59, while her HDL is a monumental 109!

I told her my rule of HDL equals your predicted age before disease. "You may make it to 109 with these numbers," I said shaking my head in utter amazement. Her ratio was a mere .54, the very best I had ever seen. "Your arteries must be like polished mirrors, because your HDL keeps them so clean," I imagined.

Normally a person needs at least one HDL molecule to clean up after three triglycerides. I barely had that with 42 HDL to clean up and get rid of my 120 triglycerides. Faith, on the other hand, only needed 20 HDL to clean up her 59 triglycerides. She had an extra 89 HDL just sitting around waiting for something to do.

"Can you loan them to me?" I asked.

THE TG/HDL RATIO: WHAT IS YOURS?

Healthy Genes	Borderline Genes	Unhealthy Genes
* Less Than 1.0	* 1.0 to 3.0	* Greater than 3.0
* Longevity	* Lower Risk of Diabetes	* Increased Risk of Heart Attack
* Lean Body Type	* Less Dementia Risk	* Increased Cancer Risk
* Preserved Brain Function	* Lower Death Risk	* Poor Response to Cancer RX
* Better Survival w Disease	* Achievable w Lifestyle *	* Associated w IR & Obesity

EASY WAYS TO LOWER YOUR TG/HDL RATIO

* Coffee and Whey before Bad Food [Sugar, Meat, or Trans or Saturated Fat]
* Intermittent Fasting [TRE] 16:8 Four Days per Week
* Strength Training
* Gradually Decrease Bad food to One Day per week [Cheat Meal]
*

FOODS THAT CHANGE THE TG/HDL RATIO [5]

Longevity (GOOD) Foods that Lower It:	Life-Shortening (BAD) Foods that Increase It:
• Wine	* Red & Processed Meat
• Coffee French	* Fries
• Low-Fat & Fermented Dairy	* Butter/Milk
• Dark Yellow Vegetables	* Margarine
• Green Leafy Vegetables	* Refined Grains
• Whole Fruit	* Diet Soda
• Olive Oil	* Heavy Alcohol
• Fibrous Vegetables like Brocolli	* Starchy Vegetables: Potatoes
• Nuts	* Creamed & Noodle Soups

Pay attention to details. Know that the main damage done to your arteries and cells is during the post-meal phase. That is when the killer microns and sugar shards are at their highest levels and can cause the most elevations of VLDL, LDL, and glucose. That is when the damage is done.

To combat this, you will want to eat smaller, less fatty, and lower glycemic meals. Always combine meals with coffee and whey preloads. For larger meals, feasts, or celebration dinners like on Thanksgiving or Christmas do what I do.

Do some light resistive exercise a few hours before the meal in addition to preloading with coffee and whey. This will prime your muscles to rapidly absorb the sugar and keep your levels of insulin and glucose low in response to the feast. If you are already eating like an Adventist with many plant-based foods, your levels will not spike much in the first place anyway.

***

Sudden Death: Your First Symptom

I have lost many dear friends to metabolic syndrome who didn't have the benefit of the knowledge that we have today. Mr. Sommers was my favorite high school teacher. He played a mean game of chess and he taught an even meaner course of tenth grade geometry. He even allowed me to sit in the back of the class playing chess on my portable pocket set so long as I did well on his exams.

Mr. Sommers was not just the coolest high school teacher. He even drove me in his Cadillac Coupe Deville to Indiana State chess tournaments, bought me dinner, and became a best friend. He helped me found the first Hobart High School chess club. His wife taught economics and made cookies each Christmas. She was a plumper version of my grandmother and very sweet. Both Mr. and Mrs. Sommers, popular teachers at my high school, were more than overweight, more than pleasantly plump. They were obese in the year 1972, a time when the obesity rate was 16% nationally. It is now 36%

Mr. Sommers also smoked. In the 1970s, roughly half the population smoked including my dad. Although my dad had great genetics and was lean and fit no matter what he ate, Mr. Sommers was more like me. He had clear evidence of metabolic syndrome. He looked like he never exercised.

One day, Mr. Sommers did not come to class. Rumor was that he had died suddenly and without the slightest warning. To my knowledge he had no history of heart disease.

We know that for one-third of the time heart disease's first symptom, its only warning sign is not chest pain. The first warning one-third of the time is your sudden death. It didn't seem fair. Seeing Mrs. Sommers dressed in black wiping away tears as she wandered the Halls of Hobart High School was difficult. How would it affect her? Both of them were in their late 40s, and now she was widowed.

Mr. Sommers has been dead now some 45 years, nearly half a century. If only he had known what we know now, that heart disease even in those with bad genetics can be avoided through careful lifestyle changes. He was cheated out of at least 30 years.

If he hadn't been cut down in his prime with a heart attack, how long would he have lived? The rate of heart disease (age-adjusted mortality rate) in 1970 was 500 per 100,000 individuals. In 2014 it had dropped to 167 per 100,000, a decrease of 2/3 or 66%.

Much of this is due to our better treatment of metabolic risk factors such as blood pressure and cholesterol. In 1971, 18% of the population had high blood pressure and only 1/3 was under treatment. More than ½ of the time this treatment was unsuccessful to control the condition.

63% of those affected were on no treatment and only 16% of hypertension was under control. Just nine years later in 1980, a government educational campaign had made astonishing progress. 56% of hypertensives were now on medication and a full 34% - double- were under control.

In the 1980s ACE inhibitors, blood pressure medications like captopril and lisinopril were FDA approved. These were much more effective than the old-fashioned ones. Today, we have angiotensin receptor blockers, more powerful with even fewer side effects, as well as a host of other treatments. Better attention and treatment of hypertension led to massive reductions in cardiovascular disease.

Concurrently, smoking, perhaps the #1 risk factor for heart disease, dropped to about 50% of the population in 1970 and 20% of the population today. Having statin medications like Lipitor made a huge difference, too. Statins were first introduced in 1987 and this led to huge reductions of both cholesterol and heart disease risk. Newer more powerful statins like Crestor can reduce cholesterol by more than 50% and are now widely prescribed and available. These account for a 22 billion dollar annual statin industry.

The combination of better treatments for hypertension as well as for cholesterol combined with a lower rate of smoking are only part of the story of heart disease. Treatments for heart disease, once it has struck, have also become part of the equation. Although the first bypass surgery was technically performed in 1960, it was not until Dr. René Favaloro developed the saphenous vein graft bypass technique in 1967 that widespread application took place. This procedure can now add 10-15 years of life to one with imminently-fatal heart disease. Byron had this type of surgery.

By 1986, the first coronary artery stents were developed. Julio Palomar developed the first balloon angioplasty, which allowed a narrowed and diseased vessels to be reopened without the need for cutting the chest open. Newer and better stents were later developed further extending survival in those with heart disease. Due to early detection, aggressive risk factor control, and effective treatment of disease, heart disease deaths have dropped 66% over the last 45 years.

Stroke with virtually the same risk factors as heart disease has dropped even more. The age-adjusted stroke mortality rate in 1970 was 156 per 100,000 people. In 2014 it had dropped to 40.5 deaths per 100,000, a drop of 74%. This drop was attributed as well to decreases in smoking, better control of cholesterol and blood pressure, and better treatment with the development of specialized stroke rehabilitation centers.

My guess is that Mr. Sommers would have lived at least another 10-15 years had he stopped smoking and gotten his blood pressure and cholesterol under control.

Advances in the treatment of heart disease have been a huge positive, but what diseases have increased since 1970? Diabetes has gone from a disease afflicting four million in 1971 to afflicting twenty-three million Americans in 2015. Diabetes more than doubles the risk of contracting either fatal heart disease or stroke. The increased rate of diabetes has paralleled the increased rates of overweight and obesity. Obesity accounted for 13% of the population in 1960 and today accounts for about 36% of the population. This is almost tripling.

HEART DISEASE ADVANCES THE LAST 50 YEARS

* Improved Prevention:	* Blood Pressure Control---ACE Inhibitors
	* Cholesterol Control---Statins
	* Non-Smoking Education

* Improved Treatment:	* Bypass Surgery
	* Balloon Angioplasty
	* Stents

EMERGING HEALTH RISK FACTORS TODAY

* Obesity Epidemic
* Diabetes Epidemic
* Metabolic Syndrome Epidemic

***

The Scale of the Problem

With the proliferation of fast food restaurant chains, comfort foods, high fructose corn syrup, and long episodes of sitting through internet surfing, gaming, and television watching, the conditions are ripe for a perfect storm of metabolic disease. Compounding matters is nighttime eating, which is thought to do the most damage.

In the U.S., the diabetes rate was 1% in 1960. Some 60 years later, and some 4,200 fast food restaurants later, we now have a rate of 10%—with another 33% with prediabetes—and an obesity epidemic. China has duplicated our trajectory in only 30 years. In 1980, China had a diabetes rate of .6%. From 1980 to 2010, that rate has increased to 11% of the population with another 36% with prediabetes. All of these people are ticking time bombs just waiting to explode with cancers, dementias, and heart attacks. With 1.1 billion people, China has about 120 million diabetics, almost sixfold more than the United States.

Percentage of Population with Diabetes

>10 %	4 %	1 %	< 1 %
* China in 2010	* U.S. in 1980	* U.S. in 1960	* China in 1980
* India in 2017			
* U.S. in 2017			

The Best Whey to Combat the Obesity Epidemic

Coffee is one of the most potent ways to prevent type II diabetes, and with the rise of Starbucks and other coffee chains around the world, it seems best positioned as the solution. Both coffee and whey dramatically lower inflammation and oxidative stress, the chief risk factors for both heart disease and cancer. Adding whey protein to one's coffee can encourage weight loss even without exercise supplementation.

Instead of insisting that people embark on an exercise program of 10,000 steps a day which they seldom follow long term, why not at the very least recommend that people restrict their screen times to a maximum of three hours per day before bed? Why not recommend that people drink coffee and whey protein before meals? Why not recommend that people restrict their eating to an eight-hour time frame each day? These are all very easy changes to make.

If Mr. Sommers could have stopped smoking, controlled his blood pressure and cholesterol, and reduced his weight with coffee, time-restricted eating, whey protein, and possibly broken up his marathon chess tournaments with periods of walking and standing, he may have been able to live a normal life expectancy – in 1971 a normal male was expected to live to 67.1 years.

Sitting and inactivity are both life-shortening habits. Faith and I personally spend 15-20 minutes three to five days a week in resistance training (RT), exercises that strengthen muscle and elevate heart rate. It is a way of building muscle and getting aerobic exercise at the same time. I limit rest periods between sets at 60 seconds. The time commitment is minimal, while the benefit is enormous.

Having fat genes is no longer an excuse for obesity, inflammation, oxidation, disease, or an early death. Know your numbers, know your risk, and do something about it today. Get on board with the Coffee Cure.

Chapter 3

THE COFFEE CURE DIET PLAN

"I feel like this eating lifestyle is one that I can keep following with no ending date." –Don M.

If you enjoy coffee already, congratulations: you will love this program. If you do not, you will want to start slow and learn to like it like I did.

Let's get started.

The Four Pillars

As I explained to Byron, the Coffee Cure Diet rests on four pillars. They are:

Pillar 1:   Coffee:

Drink 8 oz of coffee before each meal, ideally one-half hour before.

Pillar 2:   Whey Protein:

Add 15 grams of whey protein to the coffee and consume both 8 oz of coffee and 15 grams of whey protein one-half hour before each meal.

Pillar 3:   16 Hour Fast:

Four days per week. From the last bite of eating one day to the first bite of eating the next sixteen hours should pass. The goal is to practice these fasts at least four days per week, ideally five days during the weight-loss phase. These days can be in a row or on alternate days, depending on your preference.

<u>Pillar</u> 4:   <u>Resistive Training</u>:

This involves 15 minutes of RT (resistive training) four days a week, ideally five days during the weight-loss phase. This amounts to a little more than one hour a week, so it is a minimal time commitment.

The coffee can be caffeinated or decaffeinated depending on your preference. Make sure the coffee is filtered, though, as that is healthier than unfiltered. And I would not recommend more than four 8 oz cups of caffeinated coffee per day long-term, in general, for anyone. I do not recommend any women who are pregnant to utilize the Coffee Cure or drink coffee as it can cause difficulties in that group.

The whey protein can be vanilla, banana, or chocolate; essentially any flavor can be used as long as it does not contain more than 8 grams of carbohydrate per 25 grams of protein. Whey is resistant to dissolving in hot coffee, so stir it into lukewarm coffee. If you are running behind, it is okay to gulp the coffee and whey mixture just before you eat, but ideally you will want to have it 15-30 minutes before you eat for maximum health benefit and appetite suppressant effect.

The question that I always get is, "Do I need to drink coffee and whey before snacks or even small meals?" The answer is, "At the start, yes." It is good to develop the habit of drinking coffee and whey before every episode of eating. That is the foundation of the Coffee Cure Diet. For small meals or snacks, you could have one-half serving, i.e. 4 oz of coffee and 7.5 grams of whey protein. The appetite-suppressant effect of the whey and coffee will discourage over eating and retrain your habits.

The Coffee Cure program is flexible. It is designed to allow you to slowly change bad habits into good ones and slowly break our unhealthy Western dietary routine. Over the past 40 years, Americans have gone from three sit-down family meals per day to numerous fast food snacks around the clock. This keeps blood fats and blood sugars nearly continuously elevated. This leads to obesity and skyrocketing risks for disease.

We want to retrain you to eat three or four healthy meals in an eight to ten hour timeframe. Your body can enjoy sixteen hours of rest and repair without dealing with the perpetual onslaught of toxic fats and sugars. Coffee and whey do not count as breaking the fast. You are free to sip extra coffee and whey to suppress your appetite during the fast, whether it is an hour or two before breakfast or few hours after dinner. Late night coffee does not bother some people, but if you are sensitive, go with late night decaf. If you are ultrasensitive, use water and whey only; it is an excellent appetite suppressant even without coffee. Remember that by itself whey suppresses the appetite through gut hormones (more on that in Chapter 4). It can reduce calorie consumption by up to 30%.[6]

Once you get good at the third pillar, you can easily dial up weight loss by adding an extra fasting day. Conversely, when you reach goal weight, you can dial down fasting to maintain. Pillars 1 and 2 facilitate Pillar 3.

When you move on to Pillar 4, purchase an elastic stretch band, light resistance, at a place like Big 5 Sports. There should be a handle at each end and a door strap in the middle. You will want to start at five sets of 20 contractions each day. Seated band curls are easiest and can be done while watching television or even at your office or place of work during a break. These need be the only exercises that you do at first and during the first month of boot camp if it is easiest for you. If you experience tendonitis or soreness, take three days off and move to a different exercise.

Keep tension light when starting. Use protective eye gear in case the band snaps or breaks. I am comfortable with simple eyeglasses. I have a series of five different exercises that I recommend you start with. If you experience soreness or tendonitis on one side, you may continue on the unaffected side. As you gain proficiency, you want to switch to dumbbells. I personally use a combination of a heavy band for chest exercise, a light band for back exercise, and dumbbells for triceps, biceps, and deltoid exercises.

***

The Phases

Phase I: Boot Camp

Boot camp represents the first phase of the Coffee Cure program. Start by implementing Pillars 1 and 2: daily coffee and whey before each meal. Add Pillar 3, the time-restricted eating, four to five days a week. Begin with fourteen hours and progress to sixteen hours as you gain experience. Finally, add the fourth pillar: resistive exercise. Start with 100 repetitions five days per week with light bands and work up to 200 repetitions five days per week using combinations of dumbbells and bands.

You can easily increase weight loss by adding an extra day of 16 hour fast. As you progress you will want to eventually change your diet to more plant-based sources. You may also wish to work up to one-half hour sessions per day five days per week. You will want to give each body part a day of rest, so alternate workout sets. These exercises are not designed to win a body-building contest; they are to improve fat and sugar metabolism to jumpstart your weight loss. I promise you will not get larger or become muscle bound.

***

Phase II: Weight Loss

So you have completed boot camp and you are going through all the motions of the Coffee Cure. Coffee and whey before each meal, holding out sixteen hours before you start your daily meals, and pumping stretch bands 15 minutes a day. You have lost some weight, and your pants are loosening up.

Congratulations, you are on the right track. Now that you have learned how to step on the gas, it is time to learn to really drive. Imagine your Coffee Cure journey as a road trip that will transport you from a state of disease to a state of health.

Let me tell you about the cheat day and cheat meals, the icing on the Coffee Cure cake. Also, allow me to point out the speed bumps that you may encounter along the way. It is best to take a different route sometimes, so let me tell you about all the routes that I have already taken that are dead ends. These represent the keto approach: the low-carb meat-based diets in general, and processed foods.

The first road rule that you need to learn is the whole calorie myth. Although excess calories cause weight gain, weight gain from a high-fat, high-calorie diet produces a different type of obesity than weight gain from a low-fat, high-calorie diet. Overfeeding with high-sugar or high-glycemic processed foods can also produce unhealthy weight gain.

You really need more than a GPS to navigate this morass; it helps to be a physician and one like me who has researched and experienced every diet personally. There is a safe way to travel through a life glittering with tasty but deadly dishes. First, realize that coffee and whey before each meal help neutralize the health-damaging effects of bad fats and bad sugars.

Second, pay attention every time you see the words "insulin resistance" throughout this book. Read the book with a red pen in hand and circle these insulin resistance signs. Stay as far away from insulin resistance, or IR for short, as possible. "Insulin," however, is not bad on its own. We all need insulin. There is a world of difference between "insulin resistance" and, for example, "insulin sensitive." The latter is good; the former is dangerous. (See chapter 4 for more information about insulin resistance.)

To help keep you on the road to better health, I've made a list of key words and phrases below. As you read through the rest of the chapters keep these signals in mind. Green is good and these signs should be followed whenever possible. Yellow means be careful, and lower these. Red means "stay away".

GREEN SIGNALS:
- RT
- Whey Protein
- Coffee
- TRE
- Insulin Sensitive
- Anti-Oxidative
- Anti-Inflammatory

YELLOW SIGNALS:
- Salt
- Coconut Oil
- Saturated Fat
- Prolonged Fasts
- Prolonged Low Carb Diets
- Intense Endurance Training (Marathons or Equivalent)

RED SIGNALS:
- Insulin Resistance
- Trans Fats
- High Fructose Corn Syrup
- Refined Sugar
- Energy Drinks with Caffeine
- Inflammatory
- Oxidative

It does no good to hitch an easy ride in a sports car traveling 90 MPH only to crash and burn on an insulin-resistant blind curve. Going low-carb and high-fat as I once did may cause easy weight loss at the beginning of your trip, but you will pay a terrible price down the road; the price is heart attack, dementia, cancer, and premature death.

If we imagine how Phase I of the Coffee Cure fits into our road trip to weight loss and health, then boot camp represents the first 100 miles. With any new car, you will want to be careful during the first 100 miles; you will want to accelerate slowly and seat the rings while letting the transmission get broken in. Boot camp is when you make the four pillars a habit.

Imagine that your brand new car requires a fuel additive each time you gas up, and if you do not add the coffee and whey, the damage from burning the gasoline will ruin your engine before its time. Failure to add the coffee and whey will void your warranty of 80 years life expectancy.

You may laugh, but insulin resistance causes constant low grade inflammation/oxidation in your cells. The coffee contains polyphenols and the whey raises glutathione, and they both reduce inflammation and oxidation. They will help protect your engine. Never forget them.

Phase II starts after the first 10 pounds of weight loss and the addition of the RT and TRE. Once you are following all four pillars and actively losing weight, you have officially reached Phase II.

Throughout Phase II, try to have at least one day each week with no meat, not even fish or chicken. Instituting a "Meatless Monday" is a good tip to keep this up. Remember: Phase II is more than boot camp, which you can complete in just a few weeks. While boot camp represents the first 100 miles of your trip, Phase II is the first 500 miles. Phase II is the weight-loss phase and can take many months or up to a year for some.

Low carb does not always mean high-fat or high-meat, but insulin-resistant people do better in Phase I with low carb than any other approach. The trick is to stay away from saturated and trans-fats except for dairy and eggs which are okay. We will explain this a bit later. I call this the Coffee Cure Keto-Style approach. As we shall see later it is okay to add cheese, eggs, and subtract bread, meat, and junk food.

Breakfast is my largest meal of the day. After my sixteen hour fast, I can hardly wait. If I am starving at only thirteen to fourteen hours into the fast (usually around 9:00 AM) I simply drink another 8 oz of coffee with 15 grams of whey, and suddenly I lose my appetite. I can wait another two hours for breakfast. Imagine our vehicle in Phase I as a hybrid, and once it runs out of gas, it can still run on electricity, just a bit more slowly. Drinking coffee and whey while fasting will help you run on empty 30 more miles, enough to get you to your next meal or gas station. Use your coffee and whey to complete the sixteen hour fast.

Your car will start out with a maximum speed of 45 MPH, quite slow. Insulin resistance severely harms your performance. Those with insulin resistance get out of breath easily, and tire very quickly. This is due to chronic inflammation and low levels of muscle mass. Fortunately, this can be changed. Unfortunately, it takes time to do this, sometimes more than a year. With the resistive exercises, you are building up your cars horse power, and the goal in Phase II is to increase it by 5-10%. After the first 500 miles of your journey, with luck, you will have improved your engine to travel at a top speed of say 50 MPH. This is still too slow for the Interstate, but fast enough to make progress.

The problem in Phase II is that you are depriving your engine of carbohydrate fuel, and at the same time trying to build muscle–two contradictory goals. The most important thing in Phase II is not to go fast, but to lay a good and proper foundation of the four pillars in building muscle and metabolism, and learning how to say "no" to eating certain foods at certain times and on certain days.

The cheat day is when we park the car and pretend we have reached our destination. We set up camp on the beach, kick up our heels, and watch the sun go down while munching on pizza with BBQ wings. The cheat day is when we indulge in any foods we want as a reward for our hard work during the week.

I believe in two cheat meals or one cheat day per week. It is important to satisfy your cravings at least once a week and reward yourself with whatever food you desire. It will help your mental health and your metabolic switching, and it will not hurt your results. In most cases it actually accelerates your progress. Your body does not care what you do one day per week. It cares what you do most of the time. If you are a consistent on the Coffee Cure otherwise, a couple of cheat meals once a week are fine.

Sustained high levels of anything tend to make a person less sensitive to those things. Listening to too much rock music dulls your hearing, watching too much violence desensitizes one to crime, and high insulin levels desensitize your liver and skeletal muscle to its effects. In insulin-resistant (IR) individuals, muscle can lose much of its ability to absorb, store, and burn blood sugar. This blood sugar from carbohydrate ingestion then "bounces" back to the liver.

As if this weren't bad enough, the insulin-resistant liver is stimulated to manufacture even more glucose. In the normal state after we eat and blood sugar is elevated, an individual's insulin rises turning off blood sugar production.

In the insulin-resistant state, the liver ignores this signal and the glucose production switch is stuck permanently "on." Insulin-resistant individuals are carb-sensitive, meaning any carbohydrate they eat aggravates the situation by raising insulin levels further causing more blood sugar to bounce back from resistant muscle to liver, where it is converted to belly fat and where the liver continues to churn out even greater quantities of both sugar and fatty acids. Coffee and whey before meals helps fight this, as does muscle strengthening exercise (more on insulin resistance in Chapter 4).

Uncontrolled appetite, is unfortunately another reason IR is so harmful. As we fill up on food, insulin levels rise and increase our leptin levels which in a normal person turns off hunger. In an insulin-resistant person who is now leptin resistant, the hunger stays turned on, and when an insulin-resistant person cuts calories the hunger skyrockets. Mice that are genetically bred to have no leptin are obese.

In lean, insulin sensitive humans, leptin turns off the hunger and cravings. Because the hypothalamus of the brain becomes desensitized to leptin in IR, this becomes a huge problem. In people who consume a diet high in saturated fats, leptin tends not to work. I use whey protein as a substitute. Whey protein is a powerful appetite suppressant and can be used as a crutch until your IR resolves and your natural leptin starts to work again.

In Phase II, weight loss should proceed at 8 to 12 pounds per month until you reach your goal weight. The pre-meal coffee and whey will suppress your appetite while the 16 hour fasts will cause you to eat fewer calories. If you are not losing weight at this rate, increase your 16 hour fasts to 5 days per week. Make sure your carbs are below 75 grams per day. These two interventions will break most plateaus.

Phase II Summary:

- Drink a cup of coffee with 15 grams of whey protein before all meals.
- Eat all meals within an eight-hour window four days per week.
- Keep carbohydrates below 50 to 75 grams by avoiding bread, potatoes, rice, beans, peas, and legumes.
- Begin stretch-band strength training 10 to 15 minutes each day.

***

Phase III: Maintaining Weight

The easy part of any diet is losing the weight. Drink coffee with whey, eat meals in an eight-hour window, avoid simple and starchy carbohydrates while exercising 15 minutes a day with stretch bands, and then repeat. The hard part is keeping the weight off. Anyone can lose weight in the short run. Most regain it in the long term.

Even in the famous diabetic prevention study where individuals were successful in a calorie-restricted diet in losing weight, after 2.8 years 40% of the weight returned and there was no change in the progression of prediabetes to diabetes.[7]

Clearly, the official advice to cut calories and just exercise more doesn't work. The weight is regained in the long run because hunger and cravings kick in while the metabolism slows down after weight loss. Those are the two big reasons dieters usually relapse. But in the Coffee Cure we suppress appetite and raise metabolism with whey protein and resistive training (RT).

Phase III is weight maintenance. It officially begins the instant the waist becomes smaller than the hips.

Congratulations, the real work is done by the time you reach Phase III. Now it's time to add carbohydrates and substitute dumbbells or nautilus equipment for stretch bands. Increase your volume of exercise to 300 contractions per day. You will soon notice your muscles getting stronger. Like Byron, your energy will go through the roof.

The combination of more carbs and more muscle contractions will get you feeling like you are twenty again. The muscles on your frame will straighten your posture, define your jawline, and accent your waist. Your inflammation will fade as your muscles absorb more sugar and your abs flatten.

Phase III is where the focus is on muscle-building, adding carbohydrates, improving metabolism, and changing your tastes, all without really trying. Now is the time to add meatless Tuesdays and Thursdays. You will want to go three days a week without meat, even without chicken or fish. Replace whatever meat you want with beans or other legumes. For every 5% the Melbourne Australia Cohort group dropped meat and added 5% legumes (beans), their waist shrunk 3.5 inches on average over 11 years.[8]

The last one-half of the journey was the most fun for me, because I found that I enjoyed regular days almost as much as my cheat day. I started to crave bean dip. Health felt so good, and my cravings grew less and less. I looked forward to activity; chopping wood, cleaning the pool, spending the day outdoors, and keeping the computers and television off. Occasionally, I would skip the cheat day altogether.

The key to Byron's success was slowly adding and improving his muscle glucose disposal through building a bigger muscle sink while at the same time eating more protein and plant-based foods. I gradually switched Byron from eggs to avocados and tomatoes. We gradually added cauliflower, broccoli, and green beans. Most importantly, I helped Byron dial down his intake of saturated fats.

Many low carb or Keto disciples like I used to be have gotten used to chicken, turkey, beef, pork, coconut oil, and shellfish as "healthy" alternatives to carbohydrates. Nothing could be further from the truth. The studies show these are all highly inflammatory and oxidative fats that increase risks for heart attack, stroke, cancer, dementia, and diabetes. They lead, to put it bluntly, toward a premature death. Trust me; all the weight loss in the world will do you no good if you are dead.

The studies on large populations have shown this to be true. The Seventh-Day Adventists, most of whom are some form of vegetarian, live between five to ten years longer than the average American.[9] The practitioners of the Mediterranean diet have lower rates of diabetes, heart disease, and stroke.

Diabetes now affects some 10% of the American population. An estimated 35% have prediabetes and almost 50% of the population has either prediabetes or diabetes. Worldwide, there are about 425 million people suffering from diabetes. By 2045 the World Health Organization estimates this number will grow to 629 million.

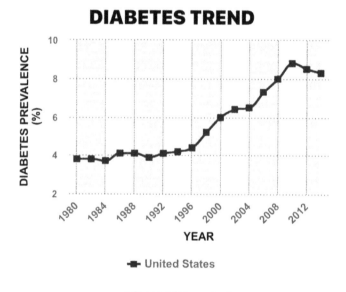

Adapted from cdc.gov

Figure 2. U.S. Explosion in Diabetes

All of this places a tremendous burden on society. The costs to our country from our diabetic population are staggering. The average cost of medical care for a diabetic patient each year is $16,750.When you consider lost productivity of roughly 90 billion dollars per year, direct medical costs of another 250 billion, and total related costs of another 350 billion, you are looking at diabetes costing us 2/3 of a trillion dollars each year.

Imagine the savings if the majority of these costs could be prevented by stopping the progression from prediabetes to diabetes with both weight loss and coffee—not just in human suffering and disease, but in dollars.

Dr. Linda Mignone believes that one way to curb this rise is to have people liberally use whey protein. She published an article in the World Journal of Diabetes entitled, "Whey protein: The whey forward for the treatment of type 2 diabetes?"[10]

I would amend this to say, "Whey protein: The whey forward for diabetes prevention!" Because if we could get everyone with prediabetes to use whey (and coffee) to stop its progression, the current 35% would never go on to develop diabetes.

The Adventist Health Study-2 revealed a rate of diabetes about 50% less in Adventists compared to our United States average.[11] Clearly beef, pork, or even chicken can be harmful to one's health. I couldn't give up meat, at least early on, so I don't expect you to. Instead, take it slowly, phase by phase, like I explained to Byron.

Substitute turkey bacon for your pork bacon. Have one day per week with no meat; meatless Mondays. Set yourself up for success. Use the refrigerator to keep your daily reminders. Once you do something daily for at least a month it becomes a habit. Once you eat differently for 30 days your taste buds also begin to change. I used to love chicken wings and pizza. Now I still love vegetarian pizza, but more than two drumsticks make me feel sick.

The most important change in Phase III is exercise, which will absorb all of those calories from any carbohydrates you might eat. The exercises help your muscle perform a miracle. It is what is known as non-insulin dependent glucose disposal. With every ten to twenty minute session on the power bands, your sugar levels will substantially drop as the muscles absorb it. Sugar that is not absorbed by the muscles shuttles back to your liver where it is stored as belly fat. Muscle exercise essentially steals fat from your belly.

To speed up this process in Phase III, I advise the use of dumbbells or heavier resistance. The longer and stronger your muscles contract, and the more times, the more belly fat you steal. No one is going to become a Hercules or body builder. Women do not need to worry about building ungainly muscles in this approach. It is simply about getting your muscles back to working normally like any thin, attractive, and lean woman would have. All the sit-ups in the world, contrary to popular belief, will not trim your waist. Building strong leg and arm muscles will.

I have been on the Coffee Cure for more than five years. Whereas I used to starve like Byron, gaining weight on no more than 1500 calories a day, I now can eat 3000-3500 calories a day without any problem. My routine involves twenty sets of twenty repetitions of light RT most days. I easily do these at home, often only three or four days per week and only fifteen to twenty minutes each session. If I am trying to get leaner or lose weight, I increase my 16-hour daily fasts from five days a week to six. If I notice that I am craving or want extra helpings, instead of indulging, I drink more coffee with whey, and I do some power-band exercises. If I am still hungry, I limit myself to one-half of an additional serving rather than a full.

In summary, the third phase of the Coffee Cure focuses on increasing the muscle contractions and weight maintenance. Weight maintenance occurs by keeping the metabolism high and the appetite in check through the use of whey protein, coffee, and muscle exercise.

In Phase III, the goal is to focus on muscle-building rather than weight loss. Increase activity in the yard, at leisure, and in sport, but above all, work your muscles. You want at least 400 contractions through 20 sets of 20 reps four days per week.

Phase III Summary:

- Keep appetite low by drinking coffee and whey before each meal.
- Focus on doing more resistance training.
- Gradually consume more carbohydrates and calories as your metabolism normalizes.

***

Phase IV: Polishing

Phase IV is where you notice at least a 20% improvement in strength and a lowered body fat percentage, to often less than 15 or 20%. Phase IV of the Coffee Cure is when my skipped heartbeats went away, when I stopped taking TUMS, when I stopped losing my keys, and when I stopped dreading buying clothes. Suddenly, everything I tried on looked great. The last 1000 miles of your journey from coast-to-coast will be the fastest. You are now traveling nearly 70-75 MPH and your engine is healthier than ever. Your inflammation should be almost gone, and what little remains is dowsed three or four times a day with coffee and whey.

Muscles will make anyone look better and younger. They stretch your face and smooth out sags and wrinkles. Not only could I see my abs for the first time in my life, on a good day I could even count them. Phase IV is where you know you have made it. Not only do you look and feel healthy and slim, but everyone around you notices it. People I had not seen in a decade all were taken aback.

"You look younger today than you did ten years ago," they say with a surprised look of sincerity.

Low levels of inflammation and oxidation will slow your aging and help keep you away from disease. By dousing the flame with coffee and whey each day, we can help a little. As the days add up, it can help much more. By avoiding processed meat, trans-fats, and sugars six days a week, we can do all but eliminate inflammation and oxidation permanently. And it shows. Health cannot help but show.

OVERVIEW OF COFFEE CURE PHASES:

	Phase I	Phase II	Phase III	Phase IV
Time	< One Month	< 1 Year	1 to 3 Years	> 3 Years
Fat Level	+++++	+++	++	+
Muscle Level	+	++	+++	++++
Inflammation Level	+++++	+++	++	+

In Phase IV, as in all phases, I encourage one or two "cheat meals" a week. This will motivate you during the week to continue all aspects of the Coffee Cure. I recommend you avoid beef and pork as these cause the most insulin resistance.

Next, I recommend increasing fish and decreasing poultry. Eggs are safer than meat, but one should strive to decrease whole egg intake to less than 8 to 12 eggs per week.

I would recommend that you strive for lower overall saturated fats, perhaps 10 to 20% of calories mostly coming from low-fat dairy. Dry cheese is a healthy option. Fermented dairy is known to lower the risks of cardiovascular disease. Some experts feel that it is due to the whey content of dairy. Others feel it is due to the increased fecal excretion of the dairy fat which never gets absorbed into the blood.

The Seventh-Day Adventists swear by it, and the studies show that it works. They have a fraction of the rate of diabetes in the general population. My advice in Phase IV is to strive to adopt a Seventh-Day Adventist type of diet, or as I will explain later, a Lacto-Mediterranean diet and lifestyle. In Phase IV you have officially reached your destination, the state of health. Congratulations.

Phase IV is about polishing. It is about consuming vast amounts of polyphenols, starting with coffee. Maximize your intake of coffee and phytochemical-rich foods. Reduce your intake of meats and saturated fats. Stay in motion. Avoid being a couch potato. Phase IV means focusing less on weight maintenance and more on strength building and getting healthier through better nutrition.

Phase IV Summary:

- Continue whey and coffee before all meals.
- Increase plant-based foods and use dairy as the main source of fat, not meat.
- Indulge in a cheat day (two cheat meals) each week.
- Increase overall movement and activity of all kinds.
- Increase [at least 50% from whole fruits and vegetables] Carbs to at least .5 to .8 grams per day per pound of body weight.
- Increase to five meatless days per week (better yet, reserve all meat for cheat days only).

***

Staying on Track

Planning will keep you on track with the Coffee Cure. It is an easy diet to follow because you won't get hungry. It is also easy because it is similar to taking a pill in terms of convenience. Instead of swallowing pills one simply drinks coffee and whey protein. One simply schedules the timing of this with the TRE. It is so simple anyone can do it. I advise all of my patients to stock up each week on the following staples:

- coffee
- whey powder
- eggs
- grated cheese
- apples
- tomatoes
- nuts
- peanut butter or almond butter

- avocados

You will want to hard boil about a dozen eggs for the week and have another dozen ready to fry or poach. Leave a note on your refrigerator door reminding you to drink coffee and whey before you grab anything to eat. Any food intake should be accompanied by coffee and whey. Also leave a reminder on your refrigerator or your smartphone to get your power band pumps done in the morning before you leave for work. Ten minutes is better than nothing, while twenty or thirty minutes is ideal.

An eight-ounce cup of coffee with fifteen grams of whey or a sixteen ounce cup of coffee with thirty grams of whey protein along with a breakfast of one or two eggs and one slice of toast is ideal. Avocado, toast, and sun-dried tomato is another good breakfast option. If you are not hungry, use your coffee and whey as a meal replacement and simply skip breakfast.

Make sure you leave 16 hours between your last bite of the day and your planned first bite the next morning. Feel free to drink decaffeinated coffee at night. If you get hungry have another fifteen grams of whey with a half cup of decaffeinated coffee. It will keep you satiated.

The hardest part is adapting to the new routine. If you have trouble, no worries. You can have two days off the TRE each week where you can eat anytime and snack late. Five TRE days a week is enough. You also get one cheat day a week where you can eat junk, processed food, candy bars, or whatever you have been craving. It will not stop your progress. If you are too busy to fit your power band routine in on a weekday, no problem. You only need to do these four days a week. Make it up on the weekends.

You can do two sessions on one day if you don't have enough days during the week to make it up. You choose which days are necessary and which days to skip, which days are convenient, and which days are inconvenient. Your body cares what you do most days not just what you do just once or twice a week. We all have kids, spouses, or significant others. We all have jobs, responsibilities, and other things to worry about besides our diet and exercise.

The good news is that the Coffee Cure diet is an easy routine that anyone can acquire. Once you get into the groove, the pounds will melt away, your cravings will vanish, and you won't ever have to think about it. It will become an automatic part of your life just as it has mine.

If you have to head out on a business trip, you will bring along your whey, apples, and nuts. You can have them on the plane along with a cup of Jo and your whey protein. I would advise against airplane food. It is filled with saturated fats, preservatives, and in some cases trans-fats. If you stay at a hotel, bring your non-refrigerated foods along. If you get hungry on the road keep a thermos of coffee or stop at a Starbucks.

***

All Whey is not Created Equal

The biggest complaint that Byron had was that the whey powder tasted awful and was clumpy. I have found that some brands are better than others. Some contain additives that I do not like. I only advise 100% whey, no creatine, and make sure sugars are no more than two grams per 30 grams of protein.

The carbohydrates should be less than seven or eight grams per thirty grams of protein. In terms of flavor, I prefer vanilla or banana, while Byron preferred chocolate with a small amount of half and half added for flavor. Half and half is acceptable in the beginning if it helps you drink the whey in your coffee. Whey doesn't dissolve well in hot liquids like coffee, but it is okay to stir it until dissolved. It won't hurt the protein or its health benefits. Some people worry the heat will denature the whey protein, but studies show that this is not the case. Whey protein has a very high biological and nutritional value even when heated.

The real trick to mixing your whey in coffee is pre-dissolving it. First, dissolve your whey in about two inches of cold water. Second, stir vigorously with a fork. Finally, either add hot coffee to this mixture, or add the mixture to your hot coffee. Voilà!

However you flavor your coffee, don't consume bottled creamers. In addition to the nutritional facts showing 25 calories per serving, the ingredients also concerned me—water, sugar, and cream. Creamer is a mixture of sugar and fat together, that deadly duo. Sugar by itself, when consumed in high enough quantities, is associated with an increased risk of heart attack by up to 300%. But studies have shown that fat and sugar when combined together are worse than either by themselves.

A dietician was once asked which food is the worst on her top ten list of "Foods to Avoid". She answered without hesitation, "coffee creamer." She explained that most creamers contain added sugars and saturated fats. Still others contain hydrogenated or partially-hydrogenated oils, otherwise known as trans fats.

To make matters worse, the labeling laws allow food companies to say "zero trans fats" even though they may actually contain .4 grams. They are allowed to round down to zero. Typically, an unsuspecting consumer uses a coffee creamer displaying a label that says "zero" trans fat. They may use two or three servings to adequately flavor their drink, confident (but incorrect) in the knowledge there are no trans fats. However, with each cup of coffee, they are consuming about one and a half grams of the deadly substance. By the fourth cup, they are up to 6 grams for the day, enough trans fats to literally kill them.

I choose to flavor my coffee with whey-based creamer. I can knock out two pillars of the coffee cure with this, and not have to worry about drinking a heart attack in a bottle.

KC Creamer*

I love my personal blend of whey protein. I did not realize that my own mix was required when I started writing this book, but I have developed it due to popular demand. I never need half and half or creamer because it tastes so good. I have found ways to make it dissolve. I have found ways to improve flavor, and I have added more vitamins and nutrients. It is now available in four flavors: vanilla, mocha, banana, and chocolate.

I call it KC Creamer as I use it as the "Koffee Cure" substitute for cream. Whey protein should be stored in a cool place as it will keep longer. In warm weather the shelf life is about three months.

Milk is comprised of 4% protein, a mixture of casein and whey. The curds represent the casein portion that gives milk its white color while the whey is the clear liquid. Whey is the healthiest portion. Studies have repeatedly shown it to be superior. Regular milk contains lactose, a sugar, which is not recommended in those insulin-resistant or those trying to lose weight. Whole milk consumption is also associated with an increase in cardiovascular disease risk factors.

Egg consumption in moderation is healthy. Studies have shown that four to seven eggs per week is associated with lower IR. Fermented dairy products are also associated with lower levels of disease and improved insulin sensitivity. Fermented dairy includes cheese and non-sweetened yogurt. The increase in the use of fermented dairy has been associated with lower risks of many diseases such as heart disease and cancer, and it has also been associated with improved insulin sensitivity.

Of all the dairy products, whey protein carries with it the most health benefits. Some scientists believe the reason that cheese and fermented dairy is so healthy is due to the whey. 100% purified whey protein together with coffee lowers the percentage of after-meal blood fats, the chylomicrons or killer microns.[12] It also reduces the post-meal blood sugar rises or sugar shards.

*These statements have not yet been evaluated by the FDA. The KC creamer or KC products are not intended to cure, treat, or prevent any disease.

SECTION II:

THE SCIENCE BEHIND THE
COFFEE CURE

Chapter 4

INSULIN RESISTANCE: THE ROOT OF THE METABOLIC SYNDROME

"Insulin Resistance appears to be a syndrome that is associated with a clustering of metabolic disorders including non-insulin dependent diabetes mellitus, obesity, hypertension, lipid abnormalities, and atherosclerotic cardiovascular disease"

-Professor R. A. Defronzo

Mandy

"Chicken nuggets and fries everyday?" I winced.

"Sometimes two servings at a time, maybe not fries, but definitely nuggets. I couldn't get enough. My record was three in a row on my birthday."

"Wow! And you only weighed 94 pounds?"

"In college I lived on nuggets and fast food. I didn't have an ounce of fat and wore a size 0. I was 5'2" tall."

"When did you change?" I asked.

"About the time that I moved from Colorado to Seattle to do my graduate work. My nose was always stuck in a book, and then over six-month period I put on about 45 pounds. I was stressed over the move and breaking up with my long-term boyfriend. And I found some comfort in my fries and nuggets."

"Did you have problems with high blood pressure or blood sugar?"

"Not then."

Mandy's laboratory studies showed a fasting blood sugar of 114, clearly pre-diabetic. She had a triglyceride level of 350. This was classic metabolic syndrome. She also had low HDL of 40 and elevated LDL of 135.

"Have you tried dieting?"

"Yes, of course. I tried calorie counting and low carb dieting. At first I lost about 15 pounds by cutting back to 1000 calories a day. After six weeks I gained it all back. The doctor told me that I should exercise more, so I joined a gym and did the Stairmaster five days a week. Still no weight loss. Then at age 30 my blood pressure and cholesterol climbed sky high. Now my weight is up to 200 pounds, and I am considering bariatric surgery. Diets and exercise won't work for me anymore."

"What do you eat now?" I asked.

"Well, I can't eat carbs, so I eat healthy fats like grass fed beef, coconut oil, and turkey."

"Any sugar?" I asked.

"I try to avoid it because it makes me gain."

"When you do lose weight, where do you lose it?"

"Everywhere except the middle. I do sit-ups, but just can't get my waist any thinner."

"Do you drink coffee?" I asked.

"No, that stuff is bad for you."

I walked Mandy through the benefits of coffee, then I gave her a list of recommendations. "Start with drinking a half cup of coffee half an hour before each meal. I want you to eat three or four times a day. No fast foods. Stay low carb. Add whey protein 15 grams to each half cup of coffee."

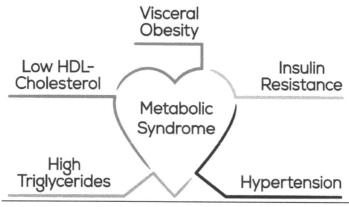

Figure 3. Metabolic Syndrome = Insulin Resistance Syndrome

Where did Mandy go wrong?

Sixty-five percent of U.S. citizens are either overweight or obese, and most have the underlying condition known as insulin resistance, or IR. Insulin resistance essentially means that visceral fat weakens the action of insulin. Insulin is required every time we eat carbohydrates. An insulin-resistant person must make more insulin compared to a thin person for the same amount of carbohydrate ingested. Our bodies will burn sugar when insulin levels are high, and we will burn fat only when insulin levels are low.

It is easy for a lean or thin person to burn fat because their insulin works well. They are insulin sensitive and don't have too much of it. The thin person stays thin easily. By contrast, an insulin-resistant person has high blood levels of insulin even when they are not eating. Even when they are fasting; it is almost impossible for them to lose fat, and they remain overweight.

35% of the U.S. population has the worst case of IR, the metabolic syndrome, otherwise known as the visceral adiposity syndrome. This combines IR with high blood sugar, high triglycerides, and belly fat, and is associated with a state of chronic low-grade inflammation. Gerald M. Reaven, M.D. introduced the metabolic syndrome to the medical world in 1988 through his now famous Banting Lecture, in which he referred to the condition as "Syndrome X." Prior to that point, scientists incorrectly attributed Type II Diabetes to a defect in insulin secretion. Dr. Reaven proved the problem was one of insulin insensitivity.

Once a person develops full blown metabolic syndrome, they are in the most severe category of IR and their risk of diseases like heart attacks and cancers doubles to quadruples.[13] Without a tool to help fight the IR, one is clearly fighting a sand hill.

Trans-fats, like the ones in the chicken nuggets and fries Mandy was so fond of, are notorious for producing IR. This can occur in as little as a few weeks. Just watch the documentary *Super Size Me* and you'll see how quickly this can happen. At the beginning of IR, the body compensates by churning out more insulin. The beta cells in the pancreas are responsible for manufacturing insulin, and they end up working overtime.

As Mandy indulged in her nuggets and fries, she was on a steady diet of both trans-fats and saturated fats. She was able to get away with this without weight gain in her teens and early twenties because the condition takes time to develop. In the first stages skeletal muscle is affected.

When insulin signals GLUT-4, an enzyme, to go from the inside of the cell to the cell membrane, the door to the cell, the muscle cell is opened and sugar enters the cell. It can either be burned or stored as glycogen, the sugar jelly. The GLUT-4 can be thought of as the doorman to the muscle. Insulin can be thought of as the doorbell.

In insulin-resistant patients, after a meal that raises the blood sugar, the insulin rings the bell, but it cannot ring it long if the person is insulin-resistant because the action is weak. The beta cells then produce more insulin, and the doorbell rings again and again as the insulin levels rise. Finally, the GLUT-4 hears the door and opens it, allowing the sugar to enter the muscle. As the disease progresses, the pancreas must produce double or even triple the insulin to ring the doorbell enough times to get GLUT-4 to answer.

Type 2 Diabetes: Insulin Resistance

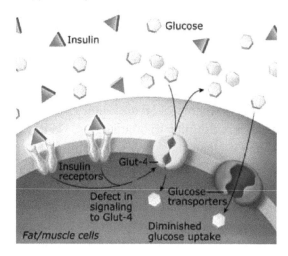

Figure 4. GLUT-4: The Doorman

While this is occurring Mandy notices nothing; no weight gain, no increased blood pressure, no increased blood sugar, nothing. This is when the condition is described as compensated. After a few years of this, her pancreas may not be able to keep up as her insulin levels continue to rise. Eventually, the blood sugar rises as the insulin cannot keep rising. GLUT-4 stops hearing the doorbell at all, and the glucose then bounces back to the liver.

The liver takes this glucose and turns it into free fatty acids. These acids are then converted to triglycerides and VLDL, a killer micron. Some of the triglycerides are stored in belly fat cells. The belly fat then releases cytokines, which cause widespread inflammation and weight gain.

At this point, Mandy began packing on the pounds. During a particularly stressful period in her life, the weight poured on at approximately 50 pounds over a six-month time period. Stress is known to aggravate and sometimes decompensate the IR. Her skeletal muscle's GLUT-4 began ignoring the doorbell almost all the time. Her liver was inundated with bounced-back glucose. Her arteries stiffened and her blood pressure increased. The soaring levels of insulin burned out the delicate liver feedback loop.

In the normal insulin sensitive state, a meal causes a small rise in insulin that normally turns off liver production of blood sugar. By contrast, an IR liver pours out glucose day and night, much of which gets converted to belly fat. After that, the IR cycle begins to feed upon itself. Little glucose will be taken up by muscle, so most is getting converted to fat. Now the liver is contributing to the problem by manufacturing both glucose and fat in addition to what is being consumed in the diet. Even when Mandy dieted or fasted, her liver continued to make sugar and belly fat. She literally gained weight as she slept.

Her muscles withered as her waistline grew. Gone was her girlish figure. In place was a heavy set apple-shaped woman. The hundred pounds of belly fat now began causing her knee cartilage to deteriorate. The inflammation caused her to develop thyroid cancer before her 40th birthday. The constant production 24/7 of triglycerides got her level up from the normal 150 to 350 and it reduced her protective HDL down to 40.

She was on the road to diabetes, atherosclerosis, and a premature heart attack. Her arteries were exposed to free circulating fatty acids 24/7 along with high levels of blood sugar. In other words, her system was swimming in a bath of sugar shards and killer microns.

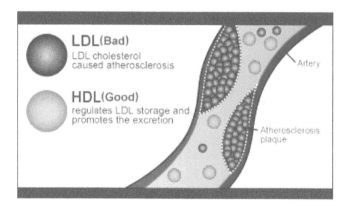

Figure 5. HDL Artery Cleanser; LDL Artery Clogger

Turning around the IR situation in Mandy is next to impossible. The longer the disease has progressed, the more resistant it is to reversal. Mandy's habits of fasting and then binging on fast foods were aggravating it. Fasting does not reverse IR or the killer micron surges, even though it may result in temporary weight loss and a fall in insulin levels. Instead, studies show that prolonged multi-day fasts can increase harmful levels of LDL, the bad cholesterol, and temporarily increase IR and inflammation.

In a study of individuals who either fasted or went on a low calorie diet, those who indulged in intermittent fasting had worse blood sugar control and worse LDL levels a year later. If an individual fasts and eats zero carbohydrates, the body produces its own sugar through a process called gluconeogenesis. Some of this is converted to palmitic acid, a type of saturated fat similar to palm oil. Even in the fasting state, the liver is churning out harmful fats and sugars, which raise inflammation levels and oxidative levels in the body.

Both inflammation and oxidation accelerate and bring on diseases. This explains why those with metabolic syndrome like Mandy have the following:

- Trouble losing weight,
- Ending up with inflamed joints, painful knees, and joint replacement surgery,
- Getting cancer,
- Developing premature heart attacks and strokes,
- Developing high levels of dangerous LDL, triglycerides, and low protective HDL.

METABOLIC SYNDROME FACTORS & RISK

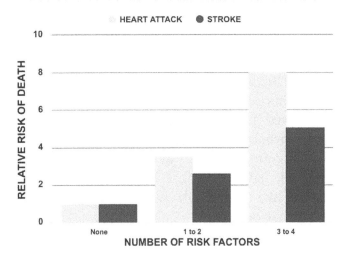

Adapted from Standl. European Heart Journal. 2005
Figure 6. Metabolic Syndrome and Risk of Death

Those with Metabolic Syndrome can be rated according to how many risk factors they have:

- High Blood Sugar. Greater than 100 fasting.
- High Blood Pressure. Greater than 135/85.
- Large Waist Circumference. Greater than 38 inches if male; 35.5 inches is female.
- Elevated Triglyceride Level. Greater than 150.

- Low HDL Level. Less than 40 if male; less than 50 if female.

Individuals with metabolic syndrome have a greater risk for heart disease and up to double the risk of certain cancers. They have up to a 400% increase in the rate of sudden cardiac death. The solution involves avoiding surges of fatty acids in the bloodstream. This means avoidance of ingesting fatty acids in the diet as well as trying to reverse the IR process.

***

All Fats are not Equal

Fats are energy-dense nutrients made up of fatty acids. Like proteins, they can come from both animal and plant sources. They are classified by their chemical structure into trans-fats (TFA), saturated fats (SF), monounsaturated fats (MF), and polyunsaturated fats (PF). They contain nine calories/gram in contrast to carbohydrate and protein both of which contain only four calories/gram. The easy way to explain the difference and the one I tell my patients is that harmful fats are solid at room temperature like lard, while healthy fats are liquid at room temperature like olive oil.

Saturated fats are generally proinflammatory, while polyunsaturated are anti-inflammatory. Fish contains high ratios of polyunsaturated fat to saturated fat, a good thing, while beef contains high ratios of saturated fat to polyunsaturated fat, a bad thing. Saturated fats are associated with increased risks of cancer recurrence. A study in 2013 showed a 5% increased risk for lethal prostate cancer and death with saturated fat consumption and a 25% decrease with polyunsaturated fat consumption, and a 33% increase with trans-fat consumption. In a similar study on breast cancer, a pro-inflammatory diet tripled the rate of recurrence. Pro-inflammatory foods include saturated fats, trans-fats, and simple carbohydrates.

Trans-fats have emerged as the unhealthiest dietary fat and one that has caused a great deal of disease. The process of hydrogenation of plant oils was invented in 1910. Hydrogenating a vegetable oil turns a healthy liquid vegetable oil into a solid toxic processed food. This led to the manufacturing of margarine, Crisco, and later other foods.

Fast food restaurants utilized trans-fats by reheating vegetable oils. Trans-fat consumption, even a few grams per day, can cause IR as well as unfavorable cholesterol profiles. The trans-fats do the worst of both worlds to the cholesterol levels. They raise the LDL, the harmful cholesterol, while lowering the HDL at the same time, the good cholesterol. They are so inflammatory that they elevate risks of dementia, cancers, cancer recurrence, heart attacks, strokes, and sudden death. Worst of all, they have absolutely no nutritional value.

The New England Journal of Medicine wrote in 2006 that calorie for calorie trans-fats are the most dangerous food substance one can ingest.[14] Dr. Mozafarrian, working at Harvard, blew the whistle on trans fats, much to the dismay of the food industry. For every 2% increase in trans fat consumption, there was a 28% increase in either cardiac death or heart attack risk. A biomarker of inflammation, CRP, was elevated 73% with trans-fat consumption.

While trans fats have been banned in many countries for a long time, the food industry in the United States resisted the labeling of foods as trans-fats and got away with keeping consumers in the dark for almost ten years. The only way one knew they were consuming trans-fats in the US was to read "partially hydrogenated vegetable oil" on the ingredients label. Your favorite cereals, crackers, and Halloween candy bars all had this toxic chemical.

In 2015, the United States finally decided to crack down. Trans-fats have been reduced, and now food manufacturers are substituting palm or coconut oil, which are both pro-inflammatory and harmful to health but continue to be found in processed foods. Trans-fats continue to be found at fast food restaurants in the form of hamburgers, French fries, etc. My advice is to stay away from them. Even if the package says zero trans fats, you may not be safe. As discussed previously, a serving can still contain up to .4 gram of trans fats and it is rounded down to zero. Always check the ingredients labels; if it says "partially hydrogenated" or "hydrogenated" anything, it has trans fats, even if it says zero trans fats.

COMMON RESTAURANT AND FAST FOOD TRANS FAT SOURCES:

- Fried Onions
- Bacon Cheeseburger
- French Fries
- Chocolate Shake

* Caesar Salad Dressing
* Honey Mustard Salad Dressing
* Anything Fried (shrimp, fries, Falafel)
* Chocolate Sundae

COMMON GROCERY STORE TRANS FAT SOURCES

- Shortening
- Cakes and Frosting
- Cream Filled Cookies
- Chocolate Chip Cookies

* Donuts
* Crackers
* Candy Bars
* Frozen Pizza

GREEN SIGNALS: HEALTHY FATS

* Monounsaturated Fats:

* Nuts
* Avocados
* Olive Oil

* Omega 3 Polyunsaturated Fats: * Fish Oil
* Flaxseed Oil

YELLOW SIGNALS: NEUTRAL TO HEALTHY FATS

Dairy: Healthy saturated due to ACE inhibition/fermentation

Vegetable Oils: Omega 6 Polyunsaturated Fats

Olive Oil Heated Not perfect due to thermal damage; but still healthy

RED SIGNALS: UNHEALTHY FATS

Trans Fats: Hydrogenated Oils or Partially Hydrogenated Oils

Saturated Fats: Processed Meats: Lunch Meats: Nitrated Meats

Saturated Fats: Cooked Meats and Fried Meats Especially

***

Am I Insulin-resistant?

If you were entering a bicycle race you would want to know if your bicycle tires were rubbing. Or if you were going to take your car on a cross country road trip you would want to know if your transmission couldn't get out of first gear, right? In both of those situations, you would have no chance of success.

Trying to lose weight with IR is no different. Because IR creates permanently high levels of insulin, it is almost impossible to burn fat. In IR the muscles don't take up blood sugar, so you will have very little energy. If you are insulin-resistant, your body will tend to convert sugars to fat in your liver and store it in the middle.

How do you know if you are insulin-resistant? Answer yes or no to the following questions:

1. Are you carb-sensitive?
2. Do you retain water easily with salty food?
3. Do you have white coat hypertension? That is, does your blood pressure go up when you are at the doctors, but remain normal when you check it at home?
4. Are you tired all the time?
5. Do you go on sugar or fat binges?
6. Do you always go for seconds and thirds at Thanksgiving dinner?
7. Do you get out of breath easily?
8. Do you gain weight in the middle?
9. Are your fasting triglycerides higher than 150?
10. Is your fasting HDL level low (under 40 for a man, and under 50 for a woman)?
11. Is your blood pressure elevated (systolic > 130 or diastolic > 85)?
12. Is your fasting blood sugar elevated (>100)?
13. Do you have polycystic ovarian syndrome?
14. Do you have prediabetes or diabetes?
15. Do you have overweight or obesity that is resistant to weight loss?
16. Have you ever been diagnosed with sleep apnea?
17. Have you been told that you have a fatty liver?
18. Have you been told there is albumin in your urine?

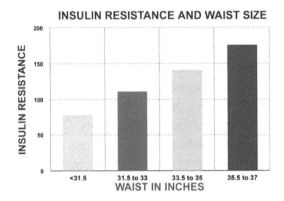

Adapted from Tabata et.al. BMC Endocr Disord. 2009
Figure 7. Insulin Resistance Increases with Waist Size

If you answered "yes" to more than three of these, you may have IR. If you have type II diabetes or prediabetes, that is a fasting blood sugar > 100, you already have it. If you have high triglycerides and low HDL and you are overweight then you already have it. If you answered "yes" to any three questions 8-12 then you already have it.

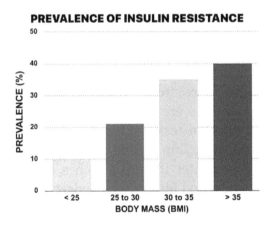

Adapted from Ferrannini and Natali. J Clin Invest. 1997
Figure 8. Insulin Resistance Increases with BMI

IR is reaching epidemic proportions both in the United States and around the world. It is closely related to obesity. The majority of people who are obese have IR.

The advice given by most traditional doctors and public health departments is to lower calorie consumption by 500 per day and then go out and exercise preferably taking 10,000 steps per day. In an insulin-resistant person, this is simply not effective. First of all, the insulin-resistant person burns sugar not fat, so they may end up burning all of their liver glycogen where they become fatigued, dizzy, and hungry, but they will almost assuredly burn no fat.

Trying to exercise with liver glycogen low is like bonking to an athlete. Bonking is when the body's supply of sugar runs out and suddenly there is no energy. They still exercise, but it is extremely difficult and not sustainable for very long. It is like asking a person without IR to strap a 50-pound back pack on and try to climb up a hill in pouring, cold rain. Sure, they might be able to do this a couple of days, but no one is going to do this in the long run.

Types of Insulin Resistance

I view IR in two categories depending upon which came first: blood sugar elevation or blood pressure elevation. There are two types: the salt-sensitive [high blood pressure], and the carb-sensitive [high blood sugar].

How do you determine which type you have?

First, purchase three items: a scale, a glucometer, and a blood pressure cuff; all three are available at your local pharmacy. You suspect you are insulin-resistant if you have trouble losing weight. However, if your waist/hip ratio is greater than 0.85 or your neck circumference is greater than 15.5 inches, you have it for sure. Measure your waist and hips at their widest portions. The waist is measured around the navel.

The next step is to take your blood pressure. If it is above 130/85 you are a salt-sensitive type. Over 140/90 means you are severely salt-sensitive. If you are on blood pressure medications, you are almost certainly salt-sensitive.

In the old days, 50 years ago, we called this condition idiopathic hypertension (meaning we did not know the cause). Today, it is known as essential hypertension. We know it is because the angiotensin aldosterone system is abnormally reactive to salt in IR. Salt overload produces inflammation triggering release of many inflammatory cytokines including tissue necrosis factor alpha, and it is also associated with neural inflammation, immune system dysfunction, abnormal heart development, and in general increased inflammation and oxidation. In short, salt-sensitive IR promotes carb sensitivity or diabetes and carb-sensitive IR produces salt sensitivity or hypertension until the insulin-resistant person has both.

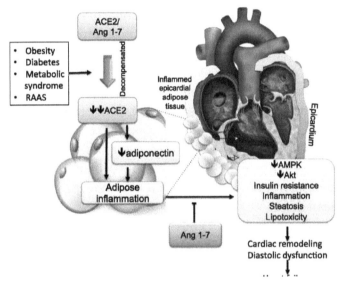

Figure 9. Angiotensin Promotes Inflammation
and Insulin Resistance

Finally, measure your morning fasting blood sugar with a glucometer. It should be done right after a 12+ hour fast and before eating or drinking your morning coffee. If it is higher than 100, you are carb-sensitive. If it is higher than 125, you are severely carb-sensitive. If you are on any diabetic medication, you are severely carb-sensitive. The blood sugar elevations trigger more insulin release. Sustained high levels of insulin trigger IR which causes the muscle to resist glucose intake triggering all the previous steps in the cycle.

If you are both carb and salt-sensitive, then you likely have the metabolic syndrome. The metabolic syndrome is the end result of IR, the culmination of a vicious cycle that can be initiated by obesity, hypertension, or prediabetes. In the full blown metabolic syndrome, one has all three.

***

White Coat Syndrome

One thing to keep in mind about blood pressure is that anxiousness and stress can affect readings. This is typically referred to as "white coat syndrome," where the patient gets nervous around doctors.

I've experienced this phenomenon myself. When I was in college, I applied for a job at Lilly pharmaceuticals. The position required a physical, and I told the doctor I was a little nervous and that it might affect my blood pressure reading. Sure enough, the numbers were the highest of my life: 165/105.

The doctor sternly glared at me and said, "Do you know what this means?"

"I don't get the job?" I guessed.

He explained to me, "You won't live long with those numbers."

Concerned, I purchased a blood pressure cuff and took my pressure daily at home. It was always normal around 120/80. That meant that I had white coat syndrome, where the blood pressure is always elevated at the clinic, yet always normal at home. I researched white coat hypertension and argued with the doctors every time that I got it checked.

Since then, new studies have been published revealing that even white coat hypertension could cause organ damage. Even intermittent elevations of pressure could adversely affect kidneys, heart, and brain. Shortly after I went into medical practice, I decided to follow my own advice. I religiously took a blood pressure pill.

Today we know that high blood pressure readings—even in those suffering from white coat syndrome—are one of the first signs of developing IR.[15]

***

Insulin Resistance on the Coffee Cure

The Coffee Cure Diet is the most effective weapon against insulin resistance. IR increases as one gains weight, but those who are still lean and have high levels of insulin are at high risk of gaining weight eventually. They have the genetic predisposition to IR, but their genes have not been fully expressed because they have not gained the weight yet.

A fascinating study by Ferrannini in 1990 was done looking at lean patients with only hypertension. The higher the blood pressure, the more IR they were. There was on average a 40% reduction in glucose uptake in skeletal muscle.[16] (As observed in other studies, IR often seems to begin in the skeletal muscles.) Carbohydrates in particular now get rejected by muscles and instead get circulated back to the liver where they are converted to free fatty acids. As we saw before, these acids then trigger elevated levels of VLDL and LDL, the killer microns. They also raise triglycerides causing a compensatory lowering of the good cholesterol, HDL. These triglycerides and fatty acids then get taken up in the adipocytes.[17]

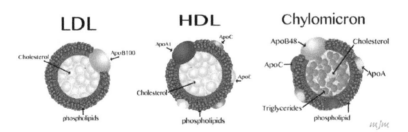

Figure 10. The "Killer Microns"

The insulin-resistant blood profile is a fingerprint or signature that typically shows normal or high cholesterol, high triglycerides, and low levels of HDL. The triglycerides and free fatty acids trigger inflammation in the adipocytes causing type I macrophages of the immune system to invade the fat cells. These cause release of inflammatory chemicals including TNF alpha and others such as interleukin-6. By contrast, the type II macrophages are found in lean people, and they do not produce inflammation.

INSULIN RESISTANCE SYNDROME (OBESE)

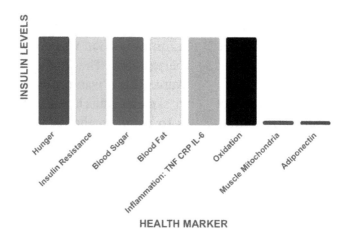

Figure 11. Relative Markers in the Insulin Resistance State

This inflammation circulates around the body increasing the risk for all types of diseases. In addition, it worsens the IR in a vicious cycle of feedback. This positive feedback loop means that the inflammation makes the muscles even more insulin-resistant, and even more glucose gets shuttled back to the liver causing even more visceral fat, macrophage invasion, and liberation of pro-inflammatory agents such as TNF alpha and IL-6. And so it continues as the person gains more and more weight, grows more and more out of breath, and has more and more joint pain. Unless they do something to break the cycle.

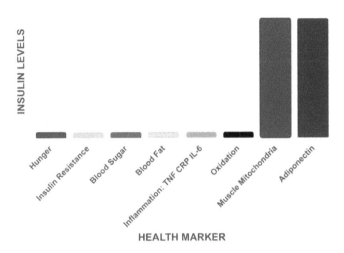

INSULIN SENSITIVE (LEAN)

Figure 12. Relative Markers in the Insulin Sensitive State

This is where the Coffee Cure comes in. Coffee contains polyphenols and antioxidants that are powerful in terms of reducing the damage from the IR. The chlorogenic acid in coffee, in particular, reduces and helps neutralize the inflammatory chemicals produced by the liver. Coffee and whey protein also stimulate the release of the gut hormone called incretin.[18] GLP-1, a specific incretin, blunts the surge of blood sugar after a meal, and the GLP-1 helps our pancreatic beta cells work by temporarily boosting the insulin secretion when we need it most.[19] This helps keep the sugar shards low so they do not do as much damage after a meal.[20]

Coffee is also a powerful stimulator of adiponectin release. Levels can rise 10 or 11% following moderate coffee consumption.[21] Studies show the more coffee one drinks, the lower the IR.[22]

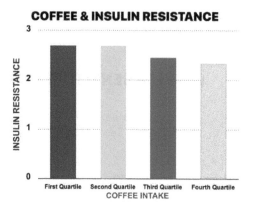

Adapted from Kim et.al. PlosOne. 2016

Figure 13. Coffee Lowers Insulin Resistance

Likewise, whey protein lowers all three culprits of the vicious cycle of IR. A 2018 study by Gao and Song induced insulin-resistant obesity and inflammation by feeding mice a high-fat (60%) diet for eight weeks. Following this, they were able to reverse all three—the IR, the obesity, and the inflammation—with alpha Lactoalbumin, one of the main components of whey protein.[23] It also lowered the MCP-1 activity, a measure of Macrophage Type I action on the adipocytes.

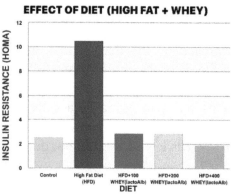

Adapted from Gao et.al. Nutrients. 2018

Figure 14. Whey Protects Against HFD-Induced Insulin Resistance

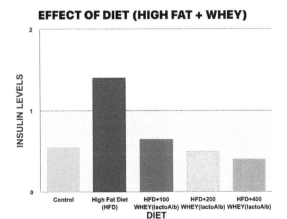

Adapted from Gao et.al. Nutrients. 2018

Figure 15. Whey Protects Against HFD-Induced Insulin Surge

As for the inflammation produced by the action of the Macrophages Type I on the mices' belly fat, notice how both of these were also reduced by the whey:

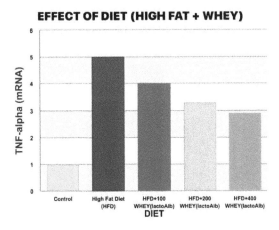

Adapted from Gao et.al.Nutrients. 2018

Figure 16. Whey Protects Against HFD-Induced TNF Elevation

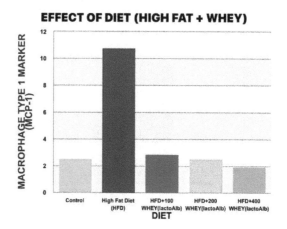

Adapted from Gao et.al. Nutrients. 2018

Figure 17. Whey Protects Against HFD-
Induced Macrophage Invasion

Finally, whey also lowered the blood sugar of the mice in the experiment:

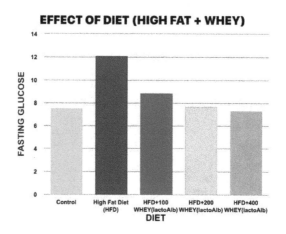

Adapted from Gao et.al. Nutrients. 2018

Figure 18. Whey Protects Against
HFD-Induced Glucose Elevation

The bottom line is that if you must eat a high-fat diet, at least drink coffee and whey protein. Whey protein can lower triglyceride levels between 20 to 50%. Coffee and whey have also been shown to reduce the levels of triglycerides and the surges that promote fat cell growth and inflammatory chemical secretion. The effect of whey protein and coffee together reduce inflammation, reduce triglycerides, reduce blood sugar elevation, and reduce the levels of both the killer microns and the sugar shards.[24, 25]

Another core pillar of the Coffee Cure, time-restricted eating (TRE), has been shown to reduce inflammation and markers of inflammation such as TNF-alpha by raising the level of the protective PPAR-gamma.[26]

Last but not least, resistive training (RT) promotes skeletal muscle uptake of glucose without insulin. This also stimulates blood flow and increases mitochondrial growth.[27] With each RT session, the muscles become more efficient, and the pump starts faster.

In short, the Coffee Cure Diet improves our blood sugar, metabolism, inflammation, and causes weight loss with lowered IR and ultimately lowered insulin secretion. It improves insulin function through improving beta cell function in the pancreas. It improves skeletal muscle blood flow and glucose uptake.

With the tool of the Coffee Cure Diet, weight control is no longer only possible, it is not even difficult. It is as easy as sipping coffee and whey, and pulling on stretch bands a few minutes a day.

Anyone can do the Coffee Cure as it takes no special will power to drink coffee with whey creamer. The power band exercises can be done any time at the home or behind the office desk. I even have watched bed-ridden patients perform the Coffee Cure. Once you dial down the IR, the weight comes off easily and stays off. Your body starts to burn fat again as your insulin levels and blood sugar levels fall. As your insulin levels fall, you become more sensitive to leptin, the normal appetite control hormone, and you start to lose your cravings.

The real value comes in lower risks of disease, less pain and a longer life. The program doesn't cost a lot other than the price of coffee, whey protein, and stretch bands or dumbbells. There is no good reason to not do it if you are insulin-resistant.

My patient told me once, "I hate the taste of coffee."

My response was, "Do you prefer the taste of chemotherapy?"

Chapter 5
THE MUSCLE SINK

"This must be wrong!" Byron exclaimed, staring at the scale in my office.

I looked at him and said, "So you are up seven pounds in three days. Have you been doing your daily band exercises?"

"Well, you know, I tweaked my shoulder, so I haven't done those for the last five days. I am resting my shoulder, you know," Byron said.

"Byron," I explained. "Remember I gave you the leg exercises and asked you to use the other arm?"

He said, "Yeah, but I walk my dog Frenchie everyday in the park. Those are leg exercises too, right?"

"Not really," I explained. "To get the muscles to take up the glucose, you need to exercise more intensively than just walking. Walking is good for you, although it is not intense enough to give you the same benefits. You can and should add it, but it is not a substitute for the muscle exercises."

When Muscles Reject Sugar, It is Stored as Fat

As I mentioned in the previous chapter, skeletal muscles play an important role in insulin resistance. Many studies have shown that skeletal muscle IR causes the sugars in the carbs to be rejected by the muscle. Instead of absorbing the sugar and safely storing it in the muscle in the form of glycogen (sugar jelly), the sugar bounces back to the liver where it is converted to fat and triglycerides. This is also where the dangerous VLDL cholesterol is produced in excess, where triglycerides and fatty acids are produced in excess, and where the HDL, the protective cholesterol, is used up.

This surges blood sugar levels and blood fat levels (the killer microns plus the sugar shards – the worst of both worlds).

Because of their outsize role in collecting and storing the sugar jelly glycogen, I like to refer to these skeletal muscle receptacles as your "muscle sink." In a healthy person, the muscle sink will be full of glycogen, ready to be used for energy whenever it's needed. In an insulin-resistant person, the muscle sink will be empty nearly all the time, leading to belly fat and weight gain.

STORAGE OF CARBS IN AN INSULIN-SENSITIVE PERSON

- Carbs--------Sugar--------Stored in muscle or liver as glycogen.
- Muscles full of glycogen fuel and function well; appear well-developed.
- Glycogen full: Lots of energy and vitality.
- Excellent exercise stamina.

STORAGE OF CARBS IN AN INSULIN-RESISTANT PERSON

- Carbs--------Sugar--------Stored in abdomen as visceral fat
- Liver glycogen full. Resistant to breakdown.
- Muscles low in glycogen. Poor muscle blood flow.
- Muscle atrophy.
- Poor energy levels. Fatigue common.

***

Muscle Exercise Reverses Insulin Resistance

Restoring muscle function is the best solution to IR. While many physicians and fitness experts sing the praises of aerobic exercise, in my personal experience I have found that resistive training (RT) is much better than aerobic in restoring insulin sensitivity for the long run. In the short run, sure, aerobic exercise helps insulin sensitivity, but the effects of an aerobic session do not last for seven days. The effects of one 60-minute RT session improve muscle insulin sensitivity up to a week later.

ADVANTAGES OF RESISTIVE TRAINING OVER ENDURANCE TRAINING

- RT is easier for bedridden or sedentary patients
- RT is superior in preventing osteoporosis
- RT has benefits to bone and metabolism which last longer
- RT produces less inflammation
- RT may be easier on the joints

Most studies have compared aerobic or endurance training (ET) to resistive training (RT). ET involves jogging, cycling, the elliptical Stairmaster, or the inclined treadmill where the heart rate increases 60-75% of maximum. This type of exercise improves cardiorespiratory fitness, resulting in cardiac benefits, benefits to glucose metabolism, and improvement in fasting blood sugars, cholesterol, and IR.

RT, on the other hand, involves contracting the muscles against some form of resistance such as weights or elastic bands. Typical paradigms used multiple repetitions of 50% of what the subject could lift maximally one time. Typically the subject did five to eight repetitions of an exercise such as a knee extension or elbow contraction, rested a few minutes, then repeated, rested a few minutes, and then repeated for a total of three sets. In such studies, RT produced improvements in blood pressure, blood fats, glucose levels, IR, and sometimes even cardiorespiratory fitness if the rest periods were short (one minute or less) and the volumes were high (10-15 repetitions).[28]

In older adults, RT is increasingly recommended as an adjunctive therapy to ET to combat the unhealthy muscle loss that typically occurs with the aging process.[29] More and more studies are devoted to RT as it appears an equally healthy alternative to ET.

It has shown a variety of health benefits in populations of patients were ET cannot be accomplished. For adults who cannot commit to a traditional endurance training program of 150 minutes a week per government recommendations, RT is an attractive alternative that can be accomplished in as little as 10-12 minutes per day and still convey enormous health benefits.

Five and Fly

My personal experience is that RT provides superior benefits to ET if done properly because of the cumulative and long term health improvements that are lacking in the typical ET or even basic walking.

When one stops walking, jogging, or cycling, there is a rapid detraining effect with loss of most if not all health benefits.

Although the benefits of an aerobic session may last up to 48 hours, the beneficial effect of a single bout of resistance exercise can show prolonged gains in metabolism and weight control, lasting up to seven days. Additionally, I find it is easier to engage in RT 10 minutes per day than making time for a one hour walk, a bike ride or trip to the gym. Indeed, Dr. Yang notes that both RT and ET provide comparable benefits, and it is not so much which one chooses as that one does something consistently.[30]

Furthermore, while aerobic benefits are lost rapidly, the effects of increased mitochondrial density in muscle persist even in detraining, and once retraining is resumed they become cumulative. Muscle mass and strength can remain for months.

Some studies, which will be further discussed later, show that RT, even after it is stopped, can produce lasting improvements in bone density for almost ten years.[31]

RT of the type I do and recommend to Byron is high volume, low resistance, and is easy to integrate into a busy schedule. It can be done in bed if one is recovering from surgery or laid up due to illness.

One study found that simply doing RT in bed, not only prevented detraining or worsened IR, but actually improved it.[32]

Some researchers have proposed "exercise snacks" in as little as a few minutes at a time. These can be as simple as seated curls with bands or light (3 or 5 or 10 pound) dumbbells; 100 repetitions or contractions would be a great snack. Other exercises can be substituted for the snacking such supine triceps pullovers, standing lunges, squats, wall slides, or supine chest presses. Bench dips, biceps curls, and push-ups are my go-to snacks. There are few things better than a hot cup of afternoon coffee to go with a good exercise snack!

I can do as little or as much as I want and in the comfort of my own home.

RT is much easier if you do not have quick access to a gym or don't feel like going out for a jog or cycling session. If there is ice or snow or sleet or rain outside, RT is the easy answer. If you are confined to an office in a high-rise building, you can easily bring your bands along and take a break. If I am in a super hurry and don't have enough time to do the full 400 contractions over 20 sets, I don't just skip it. I merely do an abbreviated version.

I perform what I call the "Five and Fly". Five sets of 20 reps, which amounts to 100 muscle contractions. It takes less than five-minutes, and I'm good for the day. I get a pump, a boost to my metabolism, and I don't need to waste extra time with exercise. You can't do that with aerobics!

Given RT's foundational health benefits in promoting skeletal muscle glucose uptake, decreasing IR, and promoting weight loss, there is no reason RT shouldn't be used by everyone (with doctor's approval, of course). I watched a special on *The Biggest Loser* weight loss contestants. Those who had regained their weight were in the majority by approximately 90%. They featured a rare case of one who kept 100 pounds off for one year. She did so by performing three hours of traditional exercises per day to maintain her weight loss. This involved a mixture of walking, jogging, doing household chores, and starting her day at 5:00 a.m.

I can't help but admire her will power and persistence, but clearly the vast majority of individuals in our society could not adopt her lifestyle. But how about this? Instead of suffering three hours per day, what if she cut her exercise down to only 15 minutes of RT daily and saved herself the other three hours. What if instead she simply suppressed her appetite with whey protein and coffee? It seems so much more practical and feasible to me.

***

Fat versus Muscle

So far we've spent a lot of time talking about the dangers of eating certain types of fat. However, the worst threat to our health is neither refined sugar nor processed fat. It is visceral fat. We all know it is the unhealthiest fat, but exactly how unhealthy is it?

Take Joyce my patient of 20 years. She can barely walk. She has had her left hip replaced, and now her right hip is bone on bone. As she struggles to rise from my exam room chair, her face contorts and reflects agony. She stands and balances her weight on her walker taking care to keep most of the weight off of her inflamed right hip joint.

She slowly makes her way to the scale. I help with the adjustments.

"238 pounds," I say.

"That is about right," she frowns.

Joyce stands 5'4" tall. She is over 100 pounds overweight.

Joyce is one year younger than me, and I have watched her suffer these past 20 years. When my knees started to hurt about 20 years ago, her hips started to hurt at about the same time. I began drinking coffee, whey protein, and doing RT. I slowly lost my belly fat, and my knee pain stopped.

Joyce did not exercise and instead of whey protein, she ate sugar. She loved sweets and drinks. She took pain pills, did physical therapy, and got one hip operation. Now her other hip is toast.

Why?

Joyce's visceral fat produced 20 years of a daily supply of inflammatory chemicals that slowly destroyed both her hip joints. The inflammatory cytokines produced by her belly fat that inflamed and destroyed joints can also damage the blood vessels in her heart, increasing her risk of heart disease. They can attack her brain, too, increasing the risks of dementia. And they can increase inflammation and risks for a variety of other diseases, including chronic infections and cancers.

What could be done to reverse or prevent this? Strategies that reduce weight and in addition improve IR seem the most effective. Weight maintenance is impossible for many. However, the best solution I have discovered is a combination of weight loss and muscle-building.

Muscle is like Health in the Bank

A 2018 study by Kim looked at 25,000 individuals Koreans and found that over a seven year period 20% developed metabolic syndrome, just like my patient Joyce. Those with the highest levels of skeletal muscle mass were compared to those with the lowest levels. Those with the highest muscle index had a 40% lower risk for developing the deadly condition.[33] Why did having increased muscle mass mean cutting the risk of metabolic syndrome almost in half?

I knew the answer to this because I had experienced metabolic syndrome personally and had reversed it, but the researchers found that fat accumulation—especially in the belly, the type produced in metabolic syndrome—is inversely related to muscle mass. That is to say, the more skeletal muscle mass one has, usually the less belly fat. The more belly fat, the less skeletal muscle.

Belly fat tends to starve and destroy skeletal muscle by robbing it of fuel and depositing fats inside of it termed "lipotoxicity."

Muscle in response fights back and can incinerate belly fat through its glucose disposal and secretion of protective myokines. It has been known for decades that excessive hormones like glucocorticoids and thyroid hormones can induce muscle loss. Additionally, diminished levels of hormones like estrogen or testosterone promote muscle atrophy.

With aging comes muscle loss and an increase in the diseases of obesity such as metabolic syndrome, diabetes, hypertension, and high cholesterol. Some studies show muscle loss averaging 1-2% per year beginning at age 50. With someone who has metabolic syndrome, the muscle loss can begin at a much younger age. The Kim study found that for every increase in muscle mass by 1%, the risk of metabolic syndrome and IR decreased by 11% on average and in some cases up to 30%.

The authors felt that activities and interventions targeting increasing muscle mass were a potent preventative strategy for lowering the risks of metabolic syndrome. Clearly, building muscle not only helps prevent metabolic syndrome, but by proxy prevents IR and its associated diseases including obesity.

FAT VS. MUSCLE

• Produces Inflammatory Cytokines	* Produces Anti-Inflammatory Myokines
• Fat deposits harm muscle	* Muscle helps burn Fat
• Associated with Insulin Resistance	* Associated with Insulin Sensitivity
• Associated with Osteoporosis	* Associated with Strong Bones
• Associated with Dementia	* Associated with Good Cognition
• Associated with Slow Metabolism	* Associated with Rapid Metabolism
• Fat	* Lean
• Sickness	* Health
• Premature Death	* Longevity

One reason that muscle is so healthy is that it promotes glucose uptake. Recall that in response to a carbohydrate meal, the blood glucose rises. Insulin is secreted and in a lean individual without belly fat insulin sends a signal to the muscle—the ringing doorbell. GLUT-4, the doorman, must hear this and respond by opening the door, thereby allowing the glucose molecule into the muscle sink.

Two-thirds of our blood glucose is therefore disposed of in this way in normal insulin sensitive people. The other one-third of glucose is harmlessly transported back to the liver where it is stored as glycogen or "sugar jelly." Zero inflammation.

When a person is insulin-resistant, belly fat is increased, insulin levels are high, and GLUT-4 simply cannot hear the doorbell pushed by the weak insulin. If either GLUT-4 is deficient or insulin is resistant, the glucose piles up outside the empty muscle sink and ultimately circulates back to the liver where it is converted to triglycerides and belly fat. Massive inflammation.

To add insult to injury, it also stimulates the liver to make even more blood sugar.

After years of this, the blood sugar stays consistently elevated (diabetes). The insulin levels remain high (IR), and the liver clogs up with triglycerides (fatty liver) while the belly gets large (visceral fat accumulation). Mice without GLUT-4 are obese and have high levels of triglycerides, glucose, and insulin.

Muscle mass and RT both have been associated with increased activity of GLUT-4. Additionally, RT promotes entry of glucose into the muscle sink without the need for insulin. In essence, most of the glucose from a meal can be absorbed into the body's skeletal muscle sinks with one bout of RT. The beneficial effects are strongest the first three hours following the resistive therapy session, but glucose will continue to be taken up by the muscles for 24 hours even in an insulin-resistant patient.

According to Peterson, skeletal muscle produces and secretes myokines, which improve metabolism and exert anti-inflammatory effects.[34] They signal pathways that are involved in fat burning as well.

Brain Neurotropic Factor is increased with RT

BDNF, a protein involved in neurons learning and memory, is increased after RT. Alzheimer patients have low levels of this. Low levels have also been found in patients with major depression, acute coronary syndromes, and type II diabetes. BDNF production is increased with muscle exercise and its main biologic effect is to enhance fat burning with a resultant shrinkage of fat deposits.[35]

Muscle is the anti-fat. Whereas visceral fat accumulation increases inflammation and disease, muscle-building burns visceral fat and exerts an anti-inflammatory, anti-disease, and anti-aging effect on the body. Ten to fifteen minutes at a time using elastic bands, dumb bells or ankle weights can make a positive difference. Strive for a total of 30 minutes a day, and remember that whey protein, as many studies show, speeds up muscle-building.

Inhibitor control (IC) is the measure of our ability to say "no" and avoiding binging. The concept of inhibitor control refers to the ability to suppress, interrupt, or delay behavioral responses towards external cues, including food. Individuals with low inhibitor control, or IC, are thought to be more vulnerable to attractive Western food that entices a person to eat.

Individuals with obesity tend to have impaired IC. Studies suggest loss of IC to be related to overeating. An interesting study published in *PLOS* in 2017 by Tsukamoto and others looked at the effect of a single bout of low-intensity RT versus a single bout of high-intensity RT. The participants did six sets of ten repetitions of knee extension exercises, one group with a light weight, and another group with a heavy weight. The control group did no exercises. Both of the exercise groups were tested with the Stroop inhibitor control test. Both exercise groups showed a significant improvement in IC. One session of 60 repetitions of RT with even light weights causes an increase in willpower.[36]

My feeling is that the more of the Coffee Cure that you do, the more you will improve, the more you will see results, the greater the motivation to continue, and the more IC you will develop.

***

The Muscle Pump

After Byron had been on the Coffee Cure Diet for three weeks, he noticed two things:

#1. He could feel his muscles "pump" quicker with RT

#2. He could keep up with Frenchie in walking, even jogging.

Why?

Obviously he had more energy because his starved muscles could finally be fed. But it was more than that. For the first time in years, his muscles were filled with blood. Like dry creek beds that flow again after a drought, Byron's muscles greeted the life-giving blood that filled his capillaries. This process is referred to as flow-mediated vasodilation.

Insulin Resistance patients have compromised flow-mediated dilation (FMD), and poor blood vessel dilation, or endothelial function. Their muscle capillary beds are blood starved, and one can see this reflected in all of their tissues, particularly their face. This improves rapidly with resistive exercises. I noted the change from Byron's original pasty pallor to the rosy hue he displayed in week three.

Improved muscle blood flow reflects improved oxygen uptake and metabolism in the newly energized and stronger muscles after Coffee Cure intervention. The person becomes more physically fit as the IR falls. They are noticeably less breathless during conversations. Study after study shows that increased muscle mass means less IR and improved muscle blood flow.

RT improves muscle blood flow as well as glucose uptake. If I skip my RT for more than a few days, I notice having to catch my breath between sentences. I simply do a five-set circuit, and then I'm good as new again!

ARTERY STIFFNESS CHANGE & WHEY

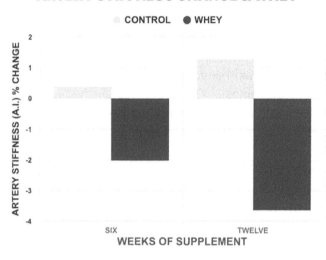

Adapted from Pal et.al. Obesity. 2012
Figure 19. Whey Lowers Arterial Stiffness[37]

I recently witnessed firsthand the effects of metabolic syndrome on fitness. Two glass installers showed up at my office to install a glass cover on a large conference room table. One was tall and lean, the proverbial tall drink of water. The other was built like a fire plug, short and stout with a large belly; clearly the cursed metabolic syndrome. Both were the same age, about 60.

The second gasped as he helped the first hoist up the 100 pound slab of tempered glass. They gently placed the glass on the table, taking care to align the computer cord grommets. Alas, it was backwards. They muscled the glass back up and leaned it against the wall. The stout man huffed and puffed and asked for a breather. The first politely accommodated him. After catching his breath he signaled the ready sign.

He really needs the Coffee Cure I thought to myself. Not just to lose weight, but to do his job. And not just to keep his wind, but to hold on to his life.

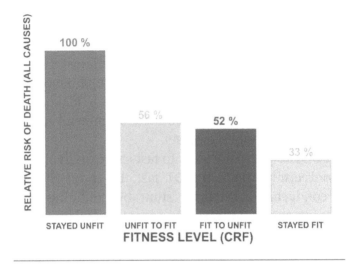

Adapted from Lee et.al. Journal of Psychopharm. 2010
Figure 20. Fitness and Risk of Death

***

Fasting

In general, we know that slower weight loss is healthier than rapid weight loss. A variety of hormones help preserve lean tissue while we lose weight. Starvation studies show that muscle can be broken down to preserve survival making this type very unhealthy.

Fasting has been highly promoted as a healthy way to lose weight by recent fat diet books. Much of this hype is based upon caloric restriction diets promoting longevity in rodents. Other studies have shown that cancer risk is lower in fasting and semi-starvation states.

However, the fact is that when a human being fasts, that means no food is being consumed. Zero macronutrients are taken in. As we have already shown, certain fats and proteins are required from dietary sources on a daily basis because the body cannot manufacture them. That is why they are called essential fats and essential amino acids. In addition, there are many micronutrients, that is vitamins, minerals, etc. that are essential as well. During a fast, one becomes deficient in these as well.

Magnesium, calcium, and phosphorus all lost during fasts can be supplied by the patient's own breakdown of bone. Some fasting proponents say that multivitamin pills can make up the other micronutrient deficiencies. Still others recommend eating lots of fat and protein before and after fasts.

While there are many ways to fast successfully, there are a few ways you certainly should NOT fast. In 2003, showman David Blaine conducted a publicity stunt by confining himself in a Plexiglas box suspended above London. For 44 days, he drank water and ate no food. In addition to fasting he was unable to move, stand, or walk, which further compounded the problem. At the end of the 44-day fast he had lost 54 pounds, a combination of muscle and fat, which represented 25% of his body weight. This was extremely unhealthy for him. He lost large amounts of vital muscle and bone besides fat. He developed re-feeding syndrome, a dangerous condition typically seen in concentration camp survivors following extended periods of malnutrition or starvation.

Due to depletion of fat muscle and both micro- and macronutrients, re-feeding in such instances produces a condition of excess insulin and high demand for phosphorus. Low mineral levels of magnesium after such a fast can cause cramps, tremors, and even seizures. Low potassium levels can disrupt the cardiac rhythm and even cause cardiac arrest. The body in such a fast can begin consuming not only skeletal muscle but also its own heart and diaphragm muscles.

Re-feeding syndrome is rare in short fasts under five days, but it is much higher in those with diabetes or IR, often the very people who seek to lose weight.[38] My patient Mandy fasted and then binged on meats and saturated fats. Byron fasted by eating only once per day also relying on saturated fats. Both remained unhealthy with high levels of insulin and blood sugar.

Contrary to popular belief, fasting also causes an initial increase in IR, not a decrease. This is the very problem that we are trying to correct to improve the ability to lose weight. Even a 72-hour fast is associated with an increase in IR in normal adults, thought to be due to blocking of an enzyme called AS-160.[39] In insulin-resistant individuals like Byron, Mandy, and myself, a period of fast can elevate IR in as a little as 12 hours. This is not a permanent increase in IR, but any increase in those who already suffer from the condition is not desirable unless, as we shall see later, one follows the fast with RT.

Before Byron began the Coffee Cure diet, he fasted 24 hours a day. Although he lost 30 pounds, he looked unhealthy, had chest pain everyday, and suffered from uncontrolled diabetes with a blood sugar of 170. Clearly the fasting approach was not healthy, at least for him. Three weeks following the start of the program with 30 minutes daily of RT, he showed substantial improvements with a drop in his blood sugar to 115, improved arm triceps muscle mass, and loss of subcutaneous neck fat. His skin color reflected more blood flow. Clearly, something was making him healthier. I believe his AS-160, which had been deactivated by his fasting, was finally reactivated by his RT.[40]

In the Coffee Cure diet, one can receive the benefits of a fast while employing TRE for a maximum of 16-hours per day only if one does an RT exercise session following each 16 hour fast. I do not recommend longer fasts especially if there is IR, metabolic syndrome, or diabetes which describes most of my obese and overweight patients. If one is free from these conditions, then with medical supervision fasting for longer periods up to 36 hours could be considered, but in any event I wouldn't advise anyone fast more than five days without understanding they may be putting their health at risk.

***

Bariatric Surgery

Bariatric surgery involves reduction or removal of the absorptive surfaces of various parts of the gastrointestinal tract.

Although bariatric surgery has been a godsend for many obese patients, it does not always produce a healthy weight loss. This is especially true in obese older adults where up to 25% of the weight loss can come from muscle.[41]

The substantial loss of muscle in someone of normal weight is classified as sarcopenia. As shown previously, muscles secrete anti-inflammatory myokines, and muscle has strong anti-obesity, anti-inflammatory, and anti-oxidative properties. The loss of muscle promotes disease by allowing an unopposed retention of visceral adipose tissue and its inflammatory cytokines.

A study by Voican looked at bariatric surgery in 184 severely obese patients. Fifteen patients of the group had sarcopenia before their bariatric surgery, while 44 more developed it after the surgery and the weight loss. Almost 25% of this group of bariatric patients developed loss of muscle sufficient to meet the criteria for sarcopenia which is highly associated with cardiovascular disease.[42]

As if that weren't enough bad news, the risk of fracture is much greater after bariatric surgery. 2,064 patients who underwent bariatric surgery from 2001 to 2009 were reviewed by Dr. Lu. Their fracture risk was compared with a matched control group of obese patients who did not get the surgery. There were 183 fractures in the control non-surgical group, but 374 fractures in the bariatric surgery group.[43] This was thought to be due to impaired vitamin and mineral absorption after the procedure leading to compromised bone health.

Chapter 6
YOUR BODY ON THE COFFEE CURE

"There are still many myths about the adverse health effects of coffee, but the latest research suggests that it is not a risky product. It increases the body's potential and protects against dementia, Alzheimer's disease, and some cancers, such as liver and colon cancer."

–Dr. Regina Wierzejska

So far we've looked at the holistic benefits of the Coffee Cure. In this chapter, we'll examine its effects on particular parts of the body, one by one.

Areas Benefitted by the Coffee Cure Components:

- Brain
- Heart
- Lungs
- Liver
- Pancreas

* Colon
* Kidneys
* Bones
* Skin
* Mind

Your Heart on the Coffee Cure

When I was a medical student, coffee was considered unhealthy. Because many people who enjoy coffee also enjoyed smoking and heavy drinking, earlier studies on its effects were flawed. They did not adequately sort the negative effects of one from the positive effects of the other. Dr. Ding and Dr. Lopez-Garcia first noticed an apparent association between coffee and lung cancer.[44] They then restricted their analysis to never-smokers only. Suddenly the associations with lung disease and cancer disappeared.

Over the last two decades, and with proper adjustment for alcohol and smoking, the evidence reveals a significant decrease in death from cardiovascular and neurodegenerative diseases with coffee consumption. There was a 15% lower chance of death for those drinking between three and five cups per day. One question was, "Why was cardiovascular disease reduced?" Dr. Lopez-Garcia and fellow researchers noticed that coffee ingestion lowered oxidized LDL. LDL is known as the bad cholesterol.

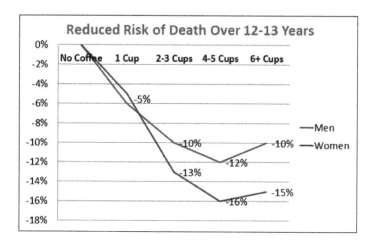

Adapted from Freedman et.al. NEJM. 2012
Figure 21. Coffee Consumption and Risk of Death

Once it is oxidized, it can react with the arterial wall, causing damage and ultimately blockage. Lopez-Garcia noticed the coffee's chlorogenic acid produced an anti-oxidant effect. It also improved insulin secretion. Both of these can lower the progression of cardiovascular disease.

What about those who have already had a heart attack, like Byron? A Dutch study looked at over 4,000 heart attack survivors and followed them for seven years. Those who drank two to four cups per day had a 31% lower death rate than non-coffee drinkers.[45]

HEART DISEASE AND COFFEE

- First Heart Attack: * Coffee reduces risk
- Second Heart Attack: * Coffee reduces up to 54%
- Arrhythmias/Atrial   * Coffee reduces risk
  Fibrillation   * Coffee reduces risk up to
- Cardiac Related Death: 50%

Dr. Mukamal, in another study, found a 50% lower death rate in coffee drinkers.[46]

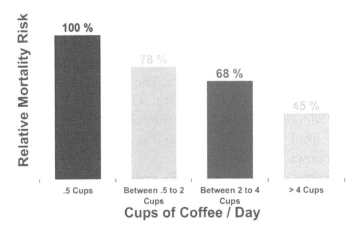

COFFEE AND HEART MORTALITY

Adapted from O'Keefe et.al. J Am Col Cardiol. 2013
Figure 22. Coffee Consumption and Heart Mortality

For first heart attacks, the best reduction was found in those who drank five to seven cups per day. Those who drank one to three cups per day enjoyed a 32% mortality reduction. Drinkers of three to five cups per day experienced a 44% decrease in the death rate.

Brown and Allgar found similar results. They noted a risk reduction in death of 21% for light coffee drinkers and 54% for heavy coffee drinkers.[47]

Clearly something in the coffee was cardio-protective after the heart attack. Another researcher, LeCour, felt the experimental data pointed to a preventative effect of polyphenols that exert cardio protective effects through sirtuins through reperfusion injury salvage kinase pathways (RISK).[48]

What about arrhythmias? Surely coffee must aggravate these. Right?

Wrong. In a Kaiser Permanente study of 130,054 adults, an inverse relationship with coffee and cardiac arrhythmia was noticed in long-term followup.[49] The more coffee consumption, the lower the rate of cardiac arrhythmia. The scientists concluded that people who drank four cups of coffee per day tended to have fewer cardiac arrhythmias, including atrial fibrillation.

But why did Byron get heart disease in the first place? Why does anyone get clogged arteries?

Because of the chylomicrons that surge and course through our blood after we eat, [50] those "killer microns" we talked about earlier. The saturated fat in a Thanksgiving dinner or a lunch at a burger joint is absorbed through the small intestine, where it forms the killer microns in the bloodstream. The "killers" attach to the artery wall and break the Teflon-like seal. Over time, lipoprotein lipase breaks them down and inflames the vessel wall, causing even more damage until eventually it plugs the artery completely. A heart attack follows.

A couple of things will help prevent this. If one consumes sufficient anti-oxidants, and the LDL never gets oxidized, the blockage will not progress. If one avoids inflammatory foods like processed and fried foods, and toxic fats, a high-risk person can reduce their danger.

Conversely, if you were born with high levels of the good cholesterol, your body will protect you. Those lucky souls born with good genetics and lots of HDL, the good cholesterol, can eat anything they want, and their HDL will protect their arteries. HDL helps clear killer microns quickly and returns them to the liver where they can no longer damage the blood vessels leading to the heart.

Unfortunately, Byron and I were cursed with metabolic syndrome genetics. We both had high levels of triglycerides, bad LDL, and low levels of the protective HDL. That is a big reason I drink lots of coffee for its polyphenols and whey for its anti-oxidants.

It is not necessary for metabolic syndrome or bad genetics to be an early death sentence, unless the individual with metabolic syndrome makes the wrong diet and lifestyle choices.

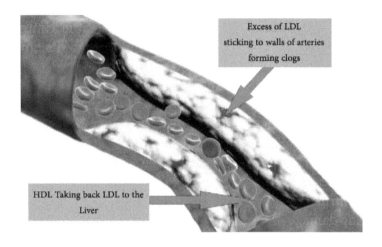

Figure 23. Protective Effect of HDL

If one with metabolic syndrome lives like a Seventh-Day Adventist, and foregoes most animal products, he can enjoy up to a ten year increase in survival, and most likely get to 70 or 80 without a heart attack.

However, if the individual with bad genetics smokes and eats red meat, there is a likelihood that the killer microns will cause a premature heart attack and death. The studies show that coffee may help delay this damage. Whey protein studies reveal substantial decreases in post-meal chylomicrons.[51, 52] Fasting also keeps insulin levels low and allows the body to repair the inflammatory and oxidative damage inflicted by the chylomicrons.

***

Your Blood Sugar on the Coffee Cure

I have a condition called prediabetes. Byron's form had already progressed to full-blown type II diabetes. It is basically elevated blood sugar. We are not alone. Almost half of the United States population has either full-blown diabetes or its precursor, prediabetes. Normal fasting blood sugar in the morning should be under 100. Pre-diabetics have blood sugars between 100 and 125. Diabetes is diagnosed when the number is 126 or greater on two separate occasions.

I bet all pre-diabetics don't drink coffee, but maybe they should. The data on coffee are clear. Coffee slows the progression of prediabetes to diabetes.

It turns out that blood sugar levels are highest after we eat causing damage to the lining of our blood vessels. This is similar in fashion to the damage that killer microns cause. Killer microns are spawned by a high-fat meal, but when we eat carbohydrates or simple sugars, we unleash different killers into our bloodstream.

Some doctors describe high blood sugar like broken glass, where the small shards cut and scrape the walls of our blood vessels as they circulate through. I call these the "sugar shards". The cutting, scraping, gouging glucose molecules create scarring of the delicate inner linings of our blood vessels, stiffening them and forming calcified plaques, similar to the stuff on our teeth that we call tarter.

Our body's natural scavengers, the macrophages, try to eat the plaques. They then bloat up to form fat-laden foam cells. Over enough time of high blood sugar a fibrous cap forms resembling a ripe, plump pimple. When it comes to a head, it bursts and a blockage forms causing a heart attack, stroke, or a ruptured aneurysm. One-quarter to one-third of the time this first heart attack results in a sudden death.

Byron was lucky the first time, but his chest pain eventually returned, and his diabetes continued to progress. When he came to see me, he was at high risk of another heart attack or stroke. The good news is that coffee can be a great tool in lowering blood sugar. Ding conducted a landmark study in 2014 reviewing data from 1.1 million participants.[53] Those who drank six cups of coffee per day enjoyed a 33% lower risk of type II diabetes.

The authors cited several coffee substances that improve IR and glucose metabolism including chlorogenic acid. Chlorogenic acid reduces glucose absorption in the intestine and reduces the liver output of glucose. It also reduces oxidative stress. Later in 2015, Dr. Yarmolinski found a similar benefit with coffee in 12,586 Brazilian adults.[54]

Those who drank zero to one cup a day had no decrease in new-onset diabetes, while those who drank two to three times per day enjoyed a 23% reduction. Finally, those who drank more than three cups of coffee per day enjoyed a 26% lower odds risk of developing diabetes.

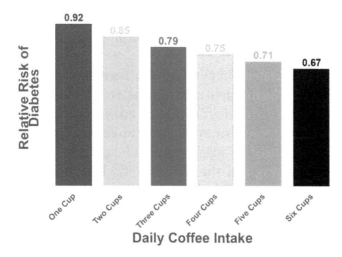

Adapted from Huxley et.al. Arch Int Med. 2009

Figure 24. Coffee and Diabetes Risk

Yarmolinski noticed there was no change in the hemoglobin A1C measure of fasting blood sugar. She felt that the beneficial effects of coffee were gained mainly in the post-prandial or after-meal phase. Yarmolinski found that coffee acted beyond its simple effects on anti-inflammation and anti-oxidation by raising adiponectin through AMPK (5-adenosine monophosphate activated protein kinase), which improved glucose metabolism.

Chlorogenic acid, the second most abundant component in coffee, reduces post-prandial or post-meal glucose levels, slows glucose absorption, and reduces liver glucose production. Yarmolinski also found that chlorogenic acid stimulated glucose transport into skeletal muscle via the activation of AMPK. She found that it didn't matter whether the coffee was decaffeinated or caffeinated; the benefits persisted. It didn't matter if the participants used sugar or artificial sweeteners; the risk reduction remained.

She concluded, "Thus, our findings support the hypothesis that habitual coffee consumption is part of a dietary pattern that is protective against type II diabetes mellitus." McCarty authored another landmark Brazilian 2006 study that eliminated any doubt about the beneficial effects of coffee consumption in preventing diabetes.[55]

In addition to coffee, protein has also been shown to improve blood sugar control by multiple mechanisms. Dr. Mignone published a study in the *World Journal of Diabetes* in 2015 proposing that whey protein could be the way forward in the treatment in diabetes.[56] She wrote that it can be used to "manipulate gut function in order to slow down gastric emptying and stimulate incretin hormone secretion," which basically means that whey protein lowers post-meal surges of blood sugar. In other words, it decreases the sugar shards.

Fasting has also long been known to lower blood sugar. The study by Sutton in 2018 showed five weeks of time-restricted eating (TRE) in men with prediabetes improved their pancreatic beta cell function as well as their insulin sensitivity—both of which lower post-meal blood sugar surges. [57]

PANCREATIC DISEASE & THE COFFEE CURE

Prediabetes:
- Coffee lowers risk of Type 2 DM up to 33%
- TRE improves Beta Cell Function.

Diabetes:
- Coffee stimulates incretins and benefits diabetes by raising Adiponectin, slowing glucose absorption, and decreasing inflammation.
- Whey improves muscle uptake of glucose and improves glucose metabolism by raising incretins
- Whey decreases post-prandial blood sugar surges
- R.T. improves muscle uptake of glucose

***

Your Liver on the Coffee Cure

Coffee loves the liver—or, should I say, the liver loves coffee. Either way, the studies show that coffee improves insulin sensitivity. The chlorogenic acid in coffee inhibits activity of G6Pase which decreases liver glucose production. Coffee tells your liver to turn off its production of harmful sugar shards. Coffee decreases insulin levels, which is a very good thing. Coffee also decreases inflammation in the liver, which in turn lowers the risk of cirrhosis.

Carrieri found that drinking three cups or more of coffee per day reduced the all-cause mortality rate in patients co-infected with HIV or Hepatitis C by one-half.[58] In a study by Freedman in 2009, coffee consumption was associated with a lower speed of progression of the Hepatitis C virus. Those who drank three or more cups per day saw their disease rates slow by 53%.[59]

Dr. Lai noticed that coffee reduced the risk of developing liver cancer by 60% and the risk of mortality from liver cancer by 90% at four cups per day.[60] Coffee is a very good thing for your liver in reducing inflammation, oxidation, cirrhosis, and cancer. It is good for your waistline as well, as it reduces de-novo hepatic glucose manufacturing (liver sugar production or gluconeogenesis).

COFFEE'S EFFECT ON LIVER

- Suppresses Liver Glucose Production (gluconeogenesis)
- Decreases Liver Inflammation
- Reduces Fatty Liver
- Helps Prevent Cirrhosis and Hepatitis

Whey protein benefits the liver in some similar ways by also suppressing G6Pase. Dr. Morifuji found that whey protein decreased calorie storage in the liver by slowing fatty acid production. It also increased muscle uptake and calorie burning.[61] Whey protein raises incretin levels which effectively lowers blood sugar.

Bartolotti found that 60 grams per day for four weeks of whey supplement in obese women reduced fatty liver markers by 20%.[62] Whey in doses under 50-60 grams per day is well tolerated and assists in reducing liver fat and sugar production. Dr. Kume suggested that whey protein is protective against the development of hepatitis and cirrhosis.[63]

WHEY'S EFFECT ON THE LIVER

- Suppresses Liver's Fatty Acid Production
- Improves Muscle Uptake of Glucose
- Lowers Blood Sugar by Raising CCK and GLP-1
- Helps Prevent Cirrhosis and Hepatitis

Chaix and Zarrinpar studied TRE in rodents and found improvements in cholesterol and glucose regulation by the liver.[64] The TRE mice were fed a high-fat, high sugar diet, similar to our

Western diet, but were only allowed access to food eight hours per day. These mice then fasted sixteen hours each day. The "anytime" fed mice or ATF mice, had classic IR with fatty liver, high blood sugar, and classic Western-diet-induced metabolic syndrome, while the TRE mice had normal blood sugars, normal livers, but had increased levels of PPAR-gamma, an enzyme known to "clean-up" the liver and metabolism. Both groups were on the same diet; the only difference was the timing of the feedings.

LIVER DISEASE & THE COFFEE CURE

Liver Cancer:
- Coffee reduces liver cancer risk up to 60%
- Coffee reduces liver cancer mortality up to 90%

Hepatitis/Cirrhosis:
- Coffee reduces both
- Whey reduces both

Fatty Liver:
- Whey can reduce markers of Fatty Liver by 20%
- TRE reduces Fatty Liver by raising PPAR-gamma

HIV Liver Infection:
- Coffee reduces disease progression up to 53%

Further, the TRE mice had improved metabolic switching. They could easily turn off sugar burning and turn on fat burning, which kept them from getting fat. The sixteen hours of daily fasts of five days per week allowed the TRE mice to combat and compensate for the damaging effects of the Western diet. In short, the TRE mice had much less IR.

***

Your Cells on the Coffee Cure

To truly appreciate the health benefits of coffee on a cellular level, one must understand its role in inflammation and oxidation.

Inflammation is nature's way of increasing blood flow, oxygenation, and nutrients to the injured area in an attempt to heal it. Inflammation in sunburn helps the skin heal faster. When inflammation persists beyond the standard healing time, it is called chronic inflammation. This can and does cause damage to our health.

Chronic inflammation in our artery walls is harmful and can trigger foam cell growth, fibrin cap formation, and the stages of vessel occlusion. Chronic inflammation in brain cells can promote amyloid plaque deposits leading to dementia and Alzheimer's disease. The most common reason people have chronic inflammation today is from visceral obesity, also known as belly fat.

The fat in the belly produces inflammatory cytokines, chemicals that create and enhance brain, joint, and artery inflammation. This leads to all sort of maladies including heart disease, stroke, cancer, dementia, and arthritis. You might be surprised to find that almost all of my patients requiring knee or hip replacements did not have any injuries to those joints. However, they were all overweight with belly fat.

CHRONIC INFLAMMATION FEATURES

- Driver of disease and premature aging
- Increases with obesity via cytokines
- Cytokines are produced by visceral fat in abdomen
- Cytokines fuel cancer, heart disease, dementia, and arthritis
- Can worsen other diseases: COPD, depression, bipolar disorder
- Associated with elevated levels of CRP

In a nutshell, they were insulin-resistant. I will never forget the knee pain that I experienced at age 45 after a workout at the gym. The squat is a great exercise for building strong buttock and thigh muscles, but my knees ached for weeks. After the exercise sessions, they popped, cracked, and throbbed every morning. I had trouble sitting for long. In med school I had been taught that this was due to osteoarthritis, supposedly a non-inflammatory condition. I had been taught that age and use naturally wear out the knee joints.

Newer molecular studies have changed this view revealing that osteoarthritis is indeed a direct result of inflammatory cytokine chemicals secreted by visceral abdominal fat cells (belly-fat caused inflammation).[65] Since I lost my belly fat and changed my diet, my inflammation has resolved.

Today, after years on the Coffee Cure, I have zero knee pain, and I use my knees everyday.

WAYS TO REDUCE CHRONIC INFLAMMATION

- Polyphenol consumption: i.e., coffee
- Avoid dietary saturated fat and refined sugar
- Weight loss
- Build muscle
- Intermittent fasting
- Lower insulin resistance

I no longer advise NSAIDs as the first step to treat knee pain, as all such pain relievers can increase blood pressure and the risk of heart attack. When my patients ask, I tell them the best way to reduce inflammatory pain is by changing one's diet and losing visceral fat. Chauhan showed that administering chlorogenic acid (coffee extract) could effectively reduce knee joint inflammation by suppressing the inflammatory cytokines TNF alpha and IL-6.[66]

Inflammation can lead to more serious problems than joint pain, however. Cancer is promoted by chronic inflammation. Those with metabolic syndrome or prediabetes are providing their own supply of cancer-causing chemicals. Everyday their visceral fat injects in them a dose of potent inflammatory cytokines that wreak havoc on their arteries, joints, and organs, dramatically increasing their chances of contracting heart disease, cancer, and dementia.

Coffee is a powerful anti-inflammatory due to its content of chlorogenic acid. Decaffeinated is nearly as effective. Hall found that coffee's chlorogenic and caffeic acids had strong anti-inflammatory and anti-oxidant properties.[67]

Whey is also healthy. It contains cysteine, which metabolizes to glutathione. Glutathione is a powerful anti-oxidant. Zhou reviewed a meta-analysis of nine studies on whey protein. In patients with elevated levels of CRP known as C-reactive protein, a biomarker of inflammation, there was an anti-inflammatory effect. This was significant for doses of whey protein greater than 35 grams per day.[68]

Eating all of one's meals in an eight-hour time frame also reduces inflammation.[69] Moro studied 35 men and randomly assigned them to control and TRE groups. The TRE subjects consumed 100% of their food in an eight hour time period. The remaining 16 hours they fasted. Control subjects ate over a twelve hour time frame. Both groups maintained their schedules for a full eight weeks. Following the eight weeks, the TRE group lost fat mass compared to the control, and the IGF-1 (insulin like growth factor one) decreased as well. This is a marker of insulin level. The changes are consistent with lowered inflammation.

Chaix and Zarrinpar's studies on mice showed profound reductions in markers for inflammation in the TRE group. In addition to coffee, whey protein, and TRE, I strongly advise a daily supplement of Omega III fish oil. All of these have powerful anti-inflammatory and health promoting effects.

However, the most important anti-inflammatory step one can take is to lose the belly fat and get down to a normal weight.

INFLAMMATION POINTS:

- This is a normal process for healing when used short term.
- Prolonged inflammation causes tissue damage, pain, scarring, and premature disease.
- Inflammation is produced by visceral fat (belly fat) leading to heart disease, cancer and dementia.
- The four pillars of the Coffee Cure: coffee, whey protein, and TRE, are all highly anti-inflammatory.

Oxidation is the other cellular enemy. It is what happens when iron turns to rust. It is the difference between plain water and hydrogen peroxide. Oxidation is what happens when wood burns in a fire. It is what occurs when your car burns gasoline or when we burn calories. It happens every time we eat. Pour water onto a sore and nothing happens, but pour hydrogen peroxide on it and see it bubble, boil, and feel the heat as it dissolves tissue, dirt, and debris. Wash your hair with water and nothing happens. Wash it with peroxide and watch it streak and turn color.

Imagine if you could pour hydrogen peroxide onto your cells' delicate DNA machinery. Instead of working like it should to create a perfect copy of itself, the damaged DNA now contains a mutation making it likely to malfunction and inadvertently create a copy error, a mutation, or a cancer cell.

Cigarette smoke is known to create severe oxidative products which produce cell damage leading to cancer and a host of diseases ranging from strokes to Alzheimer's to Parkinsonism. Even secondhand smoke, breathing someone else's cigarette smoke, can cause oxidation. Astoundingly, even third hand smoke, such as using a hotel room occupied by a smoker the previous week, can cause disease by the person inhaling the smoke-fume dust on the furniture.[70]

Oxidative damage doesn't have to come from cigarette smoke. The most common forms stem from sugar ingestion, viral infections, and environmental toxins like pesticides and heavy metals. Fortunately, if we are healthy, our bodies can easily deal with normal levels of oxidation. Oxidation in chemistry terms means a molecule has lost an electron. Another molecule gains this electron and becomes what is known as a free radical.

COMMON CAUSES OF OXIDATIVE DAMAGE

- Cigarette smoke
- Viral infections: HCV, HPV, HIV
- Obesity
- Insulin resistance
- Diabetes
- Radiation
- Air pollution

This is a poisonous cell like hydrogen peroxide that can damage anything it comes in contact with. Healthy cells have antioxidants that accept this dangerous electron back in a harmless form causing the free radical to be neutralized. It is similar to converting hydrogen peroxide back to plain water. So long as your cells have the ample supply of antioxidants with which to make superoxide dismutase and glutathione, you will be safe from the ravages of free radicals or oxidized chemicals in your cells.[71, 72]

WAYS TO REDUCE OXIDATIVE DAMAGE

* Stop smoking
* Consume anti-oxidants: whey, coffee, vitamin C, vitamin E
* Weight loss
* Lower blood sugar
* Avoid pollutants/carcinogens

WHEY'S BENEFITS

* Contains cysteine, glycine, and taurine: the building blocks of glutathione
* Whey raises anti-oxidant glutathione levels up to 7%
* Glutathione is the body's major antioxidant

When LDL oxidizes, it can destroy artery lining by embedding within vessel walls. Non-oxidized and safe LDLs, on the other hand, are neutral and do less damage, but if you overwhelm your natural defenses with a barrage of radiation damage, heavy metal poisoning, emotional stress, blood sugar elevations, or cigarette smoke, your body will not be able to maintain its antioxidant defenses for long. You will eventually pay the price with accelerated aging or premature disease.

Fortunately, most of us are not exposed to radiation unless we live near Chernobyl or Three Mile Island. And most are not victims of heavy metal poisoning unless we live near Erin Brockovich's Hinkley, CA.

The biggest secret is that obesity can overwhelm our natural antioxidant defenses through the daily onslaught of inflammatory cytokines secreted by belly fat. Metabolic syndrome patients have high levels of these toxic oxidized chemicals. Some of them are the now familiar names, TNF-alpha, Interleukin 6, etc. It should come as no surprise that the group of overweight and obese individuals now representing some 70% of the United States population is a great peril for a host of diseases accelerated by oxidative chemicals like peroxides and free radicals. What can be done aside from losing weight?

In a remarkable study, coffee was shown to have tremendous antioxidant properties. Black coffee eye drops were used in the eyes of rodents, and a poison was used to stimulate cataract lens formation.[73] Cataracts are the clouding of the eyes usually due to aging, but can be produced in rats in 30 days with this oxidizing compound. In the control group of poisoned rats, five out of seven developed severe blackened cataracts within 30 days. In the black tea and hibiscus groups, similar cataracts formed as the tea and hibiscus were not protective.

However, the group that received black coffee eye drops maintained crystal clear lenses. No cataracts whatsoever formed. The level of damaging oxidative chemicals was measured. The TNF alpha and the Interleukin-1 beta levels were markedly lower in the black coffee group indicating the antioxidants in the coffee had lowered the levels of these toxic oxidative chemicals preventing them from creating the cataracts. The reduced glutathione, the chemical that accepted the toxic electrons, was increased reflecting that the glutathione had done its job in the coffee-treated rats and prevented the oxidative cataract formation.

Thankfully, you don't need coffee eye drops to get this same protection. Merely drinking coffee is enough to help save your sight from cataracts, according to a 2016 study published by Dr. Shambhu Varma.[74] Caffeine at greater than 200 to 250 mg per day was associated with about 90% less cataract-related blindness. While caffeine is a powerful antioxidant, in the cases of individuals with PTSD and anxiety, it can have adverse effects. In those cases I would advise substitution with decaffeinated coffee. I do not recommend coffee drinking in pregnant women or those who may become pregnant. This should be done only with the approval of your physician as always before embarking on any diet or exercise program.

Although the exact mechanism is not known, what is known is that coffee reduces the disease rate in a variety of oxidative disorders ranging from heart disease to neurodegenerative disease, to multiple cancers.[75] Coffee decreases the risks for melanoma, basal cell carcinoma, head and neck cancer, breast and prostate cancer, as well as colorectal cancer.[76] Coffee drinkers enjoy lower risks of other diseases such as depression, stroke, heart disease, Parkinsonism, and Alzheimer's disease.[77]

Whey has its own antioxidant properties because it contains high levels of cysteine, glycine, and taurine, the building blocks of glutathione.[78] Whey is a rich source of glutathione, one of the body's main antioxidants. One can simply add it to coffee for its antioxidant and anti-inflammatory effects. Three to four cups per day seems to be optimal.

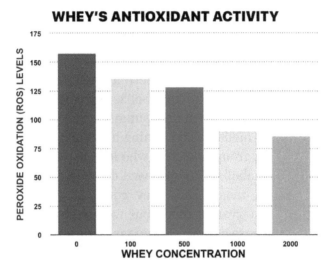

Adapted from Piccilomini et.al. Food Nutr Res. 2012

Figure 25. Whey's Antioxidant Activity

OXIDATION POINTS

- Oxidation results from byproducts of metabolism or burning fuel.
- Oxidative damage occurs to our cells when they are exposed to free radicals from smoke, pesticides, radiation, or inflammatory cytokines, or toxic chemicals produced by our visceral (belly) fat.
- These chemicals include TNF alpha or Interleukin 1 and Interleukin 6.
- Oxidation can be neutralized if one consumes sufficient anti-oxidants, like polyphenols contained in coffee or glutathione-producing substances like whey protein.

***

Your Mood on the Coffee Cure

In a study of psychological factors, consumers of whey enjoyed higher scores of vitality.[79] They seemed to have more energy than the control group who consumed an isocaloric carbohydrate drink instead. Whey protein creates a thermic effect. This means that the body must spend energy to metabolize the whey. I personally feel warm and invigorated when I consume it.

To keep your metabolism running hot, don't run out of whey. A study looked at a group of dieters who lost 30 pounds or more, and their resting metabolisms had slowed considerably, some by more than 50%. That meant that they could stay on their calorie-restricted near-starvation diets, but were still destined to regain their weight because of their slowed metabolisms.

One-half of the group tried aerobic training everyday with a carbohydrate energy drink. The other half exercised daily and took a whey supplement. At the end of six months the carbohydrate group had regained seven pounds, all of it fat. The whey protein group had only regained one and a half pounds, all of it muscle.[80] The thermic effect of whey in conjunction with exercise helps take the fat off and keep it off, so it keeps your mood up.

Michael Lucas published a study in 2014 looking at data from three cohorts of over 200,000 people. There were 277 suicides. As compared with non-coffee drinkers, the relative risk (RR) of suicide was 45% lower in the group who consumed two to three cups of coffee per day and 53% lower in those who drank greater than or equal to four cups per day.[81]

Because it didn't matter whether the coffee was caffeinated or decaffeinated, this suggested that the non-caffeinated components were responsible for the benefit. The Klatsky study found a substantial decrease in suicide risk with increasing coffee consumption. It was 80% lower in drinkers greater than or equal to six cups per day.[82]

Kwachi showed a 72% lower risk of suicide in women consuming greater than or equal to four cups of coffee per day.[83]

However, Lucas warrants that caffeine (not coffee) can trigger anxiety and panic attacks in predisposed individuals. Lucas felt that the beneficial effects might be mediated through coffee's blocking of the adenosine receptors which raises the level of several neurotransmitters, specifically serotonin, dopamine, and noradrenaline, all known to relieve depression. Therefore, caffeine can act as a mild anti-depressant that would lower the risk of depression and suicide among coffee drinkers.[84]

Lucas concluded, "Long term caffeine consumption contrary to prior report is not associated with increasing risks of cancer, cardiovascular disease, or total mortality, and overall may have more health benefit than adverse effect."

While caffeinated coffee is healthy, pure caffeine extracted from coffee is not. Many studies show pure caffeine to be harmful. Coffee contains many other health-promoting substances such as chlorogenic acid, polyphenols, soluble fiber, and potassium which can exert beneficial effects on the cardiovascular system. In a review article, Kelli Geleijnse wrote that high coffee intake (four or more cups per day) suggests a protective effect against hypertension. The risk of hypertension is greater in coffee abstainers.[85]

In a large 2018 study, Xie reviewed some 243,000 patients. Coffee consistently was associated with a decreased risk of hypertension by 2% with each one cup of coffee per day increment.[86] The more coffee one drank, the lower the risk of high blood pressure up to eight cups per day, but without the protective anti-oxidants and polyphenols found in coffee beans, pure caffeine can be dangerous.

If one consumes caffeine and sugar together, then one is asking for disease, weight gain, and premature aging as well as sudden death. Those who drank multiple so-called "energy drinks" such as college students have ended up in the emergency room with deadly cardiac arrhythmias or sudden death.[87] Between 2005 and 2011 there were 79,438 emergency room visits attributable to overconsumption of caffeine in energy-drink products. If one engages in drinking sugary caffeinated drinks, one is headed down the slippery slope of diabetes, kidney failure, and then an early grave.

The science here is uncontroverted. So, I advise my patients to give up the sugars and the sodas, stay away from processed food containing high fructose corn syrup, and stay away from energy drinks which contain added sugar or caffeine.

My patients sometimes ask me about taking coffee extract pills with added caffeine. I try to explain that it is not the same as drinking coffee. When you purify out the caffeine, you now have a dangerous processed food. Using caffeine by itself can stiffen arteries, elevate blood pressure, and cause cardiac arrhythmias. However, these adverse effects differ depending on whether the person is a habitual or non-habitual user of caffeine. Habitual users of caffeine have lower effects.

Most caffeine-related deaths from caffeine intoxication were caused by over doses of processed caffeine in diet pills or energy drinks, and most occurrences were in young patients without known heart disease. Consumption of energy drinks containing concentrated caffeine, usually with sugar, seem to be the common denominator with the caffeine's dangers. Caffeine in coffee, by contrast, is safe, and study after study has shown coffee to be health-promotive.

COFFEE VS. CAFFEINE POINTS

- Coffee is a natural healthy food made from beans containing over one thousand compounds, many phytochemicals, flavonoids, and polyphenols. It is not dangerous.
- Caffeine as consumed with the protective effects in coffee is healthy and not dangerous.
- Purified caffeine is potentially dangerous to blood vessels and the circulatory system.
- Purified caffeine, divorced from coffee, that is added to sugar (as in an energy drink) is the most dangerous form of caffeine and can cause either strokes or heart attacks even in young people.

***

Your Brain on the Coffee Cure

What effect does the Coffee Cure have on one's brain? For starters let's discuss Alzheimer's disease. Alzheimer's disease is a tragic condition where one experiences common memory lapses like losing one's keys, forgetting what one has said, to worsening symptoms like struggling to find the correct words to eventually not being able to find one's way home. It is a condition that H. Nichols has said "cannot be prevented, cured, or slowed," according to Medical News Today, February 23, 2017.

Alzheimer's is the most prevalent of the neurodegenerative diseases and has been estimated to comprise 50-70% of all cases of degenerative brain disease. It affects between 5 and 10% of persons older than age 65, and this increases to include more than 50% of those adults older than age 80. It is a disease characterized by build-up of amyloid proteins in the brain, which is highly correlated with IR.[88] The risk is increased in those with obesity and metabolic syndrome. It is correlated with increased inflammation.

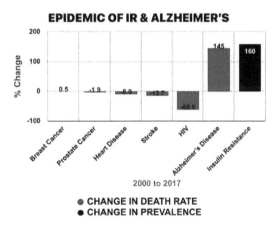

Figure 26. Concurrent Epidemics of both Insulin Resistance & Alzheimer's

Your risk of Alzheimer's disease and dementia multiplies with your level of IR.[89] Ng looked at the risk of getting MCI progressing to dementia. Those with metabolic syndrome had a four-fold increase. Those with diabetes had a 284% increase. Those with only increased waist circumference had a 41% increase. Other studies show anywhere form a doubling to a quadrupling of dementia with metabolic syndrome.[90]

Naturally, as one might expect, there are ways to lower one's risk of contracting this deadly disease. You might suspect that simply losing weight or decreasing inflammation would help, and you would be correct. You might also suspect that a diet rich in polyphenols, like coffee, would lower your risk. Again, you would be correct. It is patently untrue that nothing can be done to help prevent this terrible scourge.

Brain disease and dementia, like heart disease, are both driven by inflammation and oxidation. Thus, coffee lowers the risk of dementia. Eskelinen reported a 65% reduction in the risk of developing Alzheimer's disease in those who drank 3-5 cups of coffee per day during their mid-life.[91] In a study published in 2006, Arendash found that coffee reduced beta-amyloid protein production, one of the causes of Alzheimer's disease.[92] The Fine study, a large multi-center cohort of three European countries, found slower progression of dementia over ten years with the most benefit at moderate coffee intake (approximately three cups per day) and the least benefit at either very low or very high coffee intake (more than six cups per day).[93]

Coffee by itself was found to be neuroprotective by Dr. Richie in the Three City Study.[94] Arendash found that 500 mg of caffeine per day—the equivalent of five cups of coffee—may protect against the development of Alzheimer's disease and may be used as a therapy.

Barranco-Quintana found that coffee drinking lowered the risk of Alzheimer's disease by some 30%.[95] The beneficial effects extended to risk reductions for Parkinsonism as well. Stroke is another disease involving the vessels in the brain. Stroke kills approximately 133,000 people or 5.1% of the United States population each year. It is associated with hypertension, poor diet, poor exercise, and cigarette smoking.

Lopez-Garcia studied stroke and found a moderately decreased risk of stroke in woman coffee drinkers.[96] Lee studied a group of Koreans in the HEXA study.[97] Stroke was decreased 38% in women who averaged three cups per day. Mineharu found a decreased stroke risk in male coffee drinkers of three or more cups per day.[98]

The anti-stroke effects were similar to the anti-diabetic effects and could be explained due to the chlorogenic acid component of the coffee. This produced a decrease in the oxidized level of LDL – a killer micron – through the anti-inflammatory component of coffee. Additionally, trigonelline in coffee can also improve insulin secretion through enhancing the levels of glucagon-like peptid-1, otherwise known as GLP-1. Coffee is neuroprotective to the brain against Alzheimer's, dementia, stroke, Parkinsonism, and neurodegenerative diseases in general.

NEURODEGENERATIVE DISEASE & COFFEE

- Whey improves brain antioxidant levels of glutathione
- Whey improves cognitive function
- Coffee decreases risk up to 65%
- Up to 35% decrease risk of Parkinsonism with coffee drinking

When we look at whey protein, we find some similar benefits to the brain. Whey protein is rich in cysteine, which converts to the potent antioxidant, glutathione. In a placebo-controlled double-blinded study by Kita in 2018, 101 healthy adults with a self-reported cognitive decline showed improved cognitive performance after consuming whey protein.[99] Shertzer found that whey protein supplements decreased brain oxidation and improved brain mitochondrial function.[100]

Journel found that high levels of protein consumption signaled the ARC area of the hypothalamus to produce satiety signals, and this inhibited food consumption.[101] Long term protein consumption is associated with increased satiety and decreased food intake as well as decreased body weight in both humans and animals. This is due to the increased gut hormone secretion of cholecystokinin and GLP-1, the gut incretins.

These hormones in turn signal the ARC area of the brain in the hypothalamus to inhibit AMPK production and enhance mTOR signaling. Inflammation from obesity-related cytokines is a major driver of dementia in general and Alzheimer's in particular. Both whey and coffee are powerful anti-inflammatory and anti-oxidative agents, which help fight this. Ultimately, the reversal of obesity and the metabolic syndrome is the best way to prevent dementia.

Shortly after completing the final draft of the Coffee Cure, I read another study about Alzheimer's disease and its relationship to IR. IR of the brain has been termed "Type III Diabetes". It is similar to the cycle of IR spawned by visceral fat in the body.

This research confirms Alzheimer's disease is also driven by the same common denominator, IR, within the brain in remarkably similar fashion to IR of the muscle, liver and body.[102] This brain IR is also driven by inflammation from inflammatory cytokines, the familiar ones: TNF-alpha and IL-6. However instead of these being produced by toxic visceral fat cells, the adipocytes, they are produced by toxic brain deposits of beta-amyloid protein that reside within the hippocampus, the memory center of the brain.

The more inflammation, the more brain IR, and the more amyloid, and finally the more cytokine secretion. This spins a vicious cycle begetting more IR, more amyloid, and more inflammation, etc. Just as in the body, the process of Alzheimer's disease is driven by the inflammatory cytokines of IR. This cycle is triggered and worsened by high levels of either blood sugars or blood fats, e.g., diets high in saturated fats or simple sugars.

Remarkably, GLP-1, which is a major player in the Coffee Cure Diet's effectiveness in skeletal muscle IR and abdominal obesity, is also effective in breaking the vicious cycle of IR within the brain. When GLP-1 is increased with drugs like exenatide (Byetta) or Liraglutide (Victoza), it binds to receptors in the hippocampus. GLP-1 can also be increased naturally with coffee and whey.

GLP-1 activation in the brain can restore neurogenesis (forming new neurons), and prevent cell death.[103] This improves memory and learning. GLP-1 action in the brain also decreases neuroinflammation and reduces beta-amyloid plaque burden. GLP-1 spins the brain IR dial backwards. Keep in mind that in addition to generating the growth of new neurons in the brain, the GLP-1 helps increase pancreatic beta cell mass in the body.[104] It helps regrow pancreatic tissue.

While I frequently misplaced my car keys fifteen years ago, I have this problem much less today. Perhaps it is the GLP-1 that I naturally increased with my steady diet of coffee, whey and dairy protein. There is now an all-out research push for the rapid development of FDA-approved GLP-1 raising drugs. Some of the existing ones have not been popular as patients don't like the nausea and vomiting, the most common side effects, while other patients don't like having to inject themselves as most cannot be taken orally. In the meantime, I continue to raise my GLP-1 levels naturally and keep both my IR and body fat levels low with the Coffee Cure, all without side effects.

***

Your Bones on the Coffee Cure

To better understand the benefits of the Coffee Cure on bone structure and the risks of more drastic measures, I want to tell you about my patient Nan.

A nearly 70 year old woman, Nan desperately want to get bariatric surgery to help her weight loss, but her insurance would not cover the procedure unless she *gained* even more weight first. A month after I'd last seen her, Nan was already up 20 pounds. Her blood pressure was up to 170/100.

"Nan, your blood pressure is terrible," I told her. "How do you feel?"

"I am excited about getting the operation," she smiled.

The next month she came in wearing a Muumuu and up to 205 pounds. Her face was bloated.

"How do you feel today?" I asked.

"I have had a headache for days that won't quit. They have doubled my blood pressure medication, but I am on the schedule for July 10th."

"If you live that long," I deadpanned.

The next month she had the surgery, and when I saw her next she was all smiles. This was three months post-op.

"Back down to 175 pounds," she proudly announced.

"But what is the splint on your right arm for?"

"Oh, I messed my arm up. I fell and broke it. It hurts like hell."

Fractures are a common occurrence following bariatric surgery.[105] The studies are clear that bariatric surgery increases the risks of long-bone fractures in both men and women. For that matter, the studies are pretty uniform that some bone is lost in calorie restriction diets without exercise. When the weight is lost without caloric restriction, but through exercise, we don't see the bone loss.

Starvation and severe, rapid weight loss is associated with bone loss. Prolonged fasting is associated with bone loss, and this is worse as we get older. It is a big reason that I limit my patients to only 16-hour TRE-like fasts. Other studies show that the bone loss occurs after weight-loss diets and often does not correct following the inevitable weight regain. The lost bone does not magically return. Therefore, it is best to avoid diet-related bone loss in the first place.

In all phases of the Coffee Cure Diet, there is no required caloric restriction. The weight loss is accomplished mainly by timed eight-hour feedings which usually results in about 20% fewer calories voluntarily taken in.[106] The thermic and satiety effects of whey further burn and save calories. Although earlier studies on coffee were associated with some research findings showing some osteoporosis at high intakes (eight or more cups per day), the recent studies are almost universally positive of coffee's beneficial effect on bone.

The Korean study showed increased bone density associated with increasing cups of coffee per day.[107] Whey protein is also associated with increased bone density in animal studies. Time-restricted eating is associated with increased activity of PPAR-gamma, which activates the RAN pathway leading to increased bone formation. RT promotes both muscle and bone health. Why is this important?

Because, fracture risk as we age is associated with mortality. The greater the risk of fracture, the shorter the life.

Bone is a dynamic tissue. It is constantly being formed and broken down everyday. It is kind of like having the bathtub filling with water while the drain is open at the same time. If you increase the rate of filling-osteoblast formation, the tub gets fuller and the bone gets denser. If you slow the rate of drainage—make the drain smaller—you conserve water in the tub or bone density in the body.

Blast means bone building. Clast means bone cutting down. Coffee promotes osteoblast formation through chlorogenic acid. Patients with metabolic syndrome or IR have high levels of inflammatory cytokines secreted by belly fat specifically in the form of levels of TNF alpha and IL-6. These are associated with increased osteoclastic (breakdown of bone) activity and decreased osteoblastic (building of bone) action. By reducing inflammation with chlorogenic acid, coffee helps prevent bone loss.

Patients with bariatric surgery often lose significant bone and muscle. They often develop permanent malabsorption syndromes that impair nutrient absorption. Although they picture themselves becoming smiling, fit, and carefree individuals following the surgery, the reality is often much different.

That was what happened to Nan. A year after the surgery, she came to see me complaining about increased pain and chronic nausea. She had no energy and couldn't exercise, resulting in further muscle and bone loss. Her doctors would not allow her to eat healthy fruits and vegetables as they had too much fiber and mass for her surgically-shrunken stomach. Nan is now sentenced to a lifetime of unhealthy food.

I have other bariatric patients who did not lose the bone and muscle that Nan did. Young patients can do much better with little or no bone loss. However, the situation is not hopeless for Nan. She can absolutely turn her situation around with dedication to a daily RT program, supplementation with vitamin D, calcium, and building muscle. And of course, yes, drinking coffee and whey protein. She could have done all of this in the first place without getting the surgery.

OSTEOPOROSIS

- Modest coffee dinking can reduce risk up to 36% [Korean Study]
- RT strengthens bone
- TRE increases PPAR-gamma which promotes bone health
- Whey and RT together can improve bone density

***

Your Kidneys on the Coffee Cure

"I can eat a Cobb salad and gain seven pounds," remarked Byron when he started the Coffee Cure.

"It is probably mostly water," I reassured him.

How true that is. When Faith eats a Cobb salad, she doesn't gain weight or retain water. So, why does Byron? The answer has to do with IR and the RAAS (short for the renin angiotensin aldosterone system) in the kidneys. IR causes an increase in angiotensin-II and aldosterone, the two main culprits; they both raise blood pressure and cause sodium and water retention and unfortunately cause more obesity and more IR.

Once you develop a little IR or belly fat, this triggers the kidneys to make more of the hormone called renin. This is converted to angiotensin-II, a potent vasoconstrictor. This also causes secretion of aldosterone from the adrenal glands, which cause the kidneys to retain sodium and water.

Byron retained seven pounds of water because his IR caused an overreaction and overproduction of angiotensin-II and aldosterone in response to the sodium and fatty meats in the Cobb salad. In addition to harmlessly retaining water, his blood pressure increased and put him at high risk for a second heart attack.

A person like Faith, without IR, would have no increase in angiotensin-II or aldosterone and would neither retain water nor experience high blood pressure. The other problem is that angiotensin-II (ANGI-II) reduces blood flow to the muscle. It prevents GLUT-4 from answering the door to insulin's doorbell ring.

THE KIDNEYS IN INSULIN RESISTANCE

- Insulin resistance stimulates kidneys to produce renin
- Renin transforms to angiotensin
- Angiotensin + ACE enzyme converts to angiotensin II
- Angiotensin II raises blood pressure/constricts blood vessels
- Angiotensin II stimulates adrenals to release aldosterone
- Angiotensin II causes fat cells to grow
- Aldosterone causes water/salt retention and weight gain
- Aldosterone increases inflammation in heart and body
- Aldosterone increases insulin resistance

WHEY BLOCKS ANGIOTENSIN CONVERSION

- Whey is a natural ACE enzyme inhibitor
- Whey helps prevent the conversion of angiotensin to angiotensin II
- Whey helps break the kidney insulin resistance cycle
- Whey can be taken in cheese or as supplement

Are you seeing a pattern here? IR closes the muscle sink's door to fuel and blood flow. The ANGI-II also causes belly fat cells to multiply and grow. It is clear that ANGI-II plays a major role along with sugar and fat in promoting and progressing IR. ANGI-II causes the belly to get fatter and the arm and leg muscles to wither.

The more belly fat and obesity the more ANGI-II. Left unchecked it creates a vicious cycle of increased IR leading to increased ANGI-II leading to increased fat cells leading to more ANGI-II leading to worsened IR and so forth.

What is the solution? Break the cycle. Studies show that ANGI-II converting enzyme ACE blockers reduce IR.[108] They cause weight loss. They lower blood pressure. They slow the progression of prediabetes to diabetes by 25%. Such blockers include ARBs (shorthand for angiotensin receptor blockers) like the medicine Ibersartan, the one I take.

ACE inhibitors or angiotensin-converting enzyme inhibitors include prescription medications like lisinopril and captopril. However, prescribed medications can also produce side effects. They can impair kidney function and cause chronic coughing and other adverse issues.

Did you know that whey protein is a natural ACE inhibitor? It can lower blood pressure based on many studies of up to 2-5 points.[109] A 2-5 point blood pressure decrease translates into a 15% reduction in cardiovascular disease events like heart attacks.

Some types of whey protein are more effective in this regard. A study showed that whey protein derived from goat milk inhibited ACE to a similar degree as lisinopril and captopril, but without the side effects of taking these prescribed drugs.

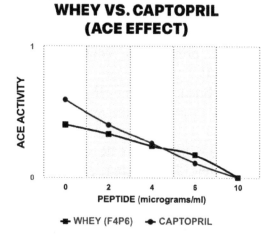

Adapted from Ibrahim et.al. J Adv Rev. 2017

Figure 27. Whey Lowers Blood Pressure

Whey protein is known to be anti-inflammatory and anti-oxidative as well as anti-diabetic. It is a major way on a daily basis to impact and block your overactive angiotensin renin system if you are suffering from insulin-resistant obesity.

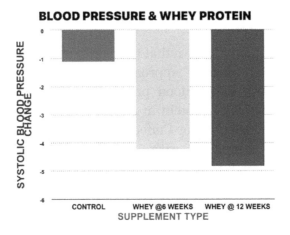

Adapted from Pal et.al. Obesity. 2012
Figure 28. Blood Pressure and Whey Supplement

In Phase IV of the Coffee Cure, I recommend adopting a lacto-ovo-vegetarian diet. Fermented dairy products like cheese are loaded with whey proteins and are healthy for those with varying degrees of IR, ranging from lean but IR, to pre-diabetic, to diabetic, to full-blown metabolic syndrome with high triglycerides, low HDL, and hypertension.

KIDNEY DISEASE & THE COFFEE CURE

- Coffee hydrates which helps lower aldosterone levels
- Whey blocks angiotensin-converting enzyme, ACE, which lowers blood pressure
- Whey reduces insulin resistance up to 25%
- Coffee's chlorogenic acid reduces I.R. via the RAAS pathway
- RT lowers blood pressure long term
- Whey protein improves artery elasticity

A recent study looked at a "high-fat" DASH diet and found improved cholesterol levels and lower blood pressures in those with the high-fat version of DASH.[110] The interesting thing is that high-fat in this program meant substituting meats with dairy. Those in the study benefited from the dairy protein's whey content. The whey had a beneficial effect on the angiotensin system which lowered blood pressures.

It has been long known that the heavily recommended DASH—shorthand for dietary approaches to stop hypertension—is associated with lower blood pressures. My feeling is that it is because of the dairy protein in addition to fruits and vegetables. Rather than DASH, go for Coffee Cure Phase III and a Lacto-ovo-vegetarian approach with supplemental whey protein. Alternatively, one can employ the Mediterranean diet with added whey, dairy, and eggs, the newly coined Lacto-Mediterranean diet. More on this in Chapter 9.

What about coffee? You might suspect that it has some sort of beneficial effect on the harmful over-reactive angiotensin system. You would be correct. Coffee's caffeic acid is a natural phytochemical. Caffeic acid itself is a weak renin (parent of ANGI-II) derivative. But compound-22 is 47 times stronger and is also a potent modulator of aldosterone production.[111]

In a group of mice subjected to two hours a day of stress through restraint, IR was produced. The stress from the restraints produced a full-blown IR syndrome. Caffeic acid reduced the IR in these mice by reducing inflammation through the renin angiotensin pathway.[112]

Finally, time-restricted eating reduces inflammatory cytokines which in turn reduces stimulation of the renin angiotensin system. Studies show that those individuals with sleep disorders or those who engage in nighttime shift work have greater hypertension. This is due to abnormal stimulation of the RAAS. In the Coffee Cure, I encourage individuals to adopt normal sleep/wake times.

Before I discovered the Coffee Cure Program, I personally suffered from all the ravages of the metabolic syndrome. I noticed skipped heartbeats that so frightened me that I made an appointment with the cardiologist to get tested.

"You are fine," he would say. But even as I lost my belly fat and got healthy, I would still notice occasional spells of these every week or so. Your heart jumping in your chest is considered an arrhythmia. Most of the time in someone my age, it is due to a common condition called atrial fibrillation. Common, but far from harmless. This has unfortunately become a national epidemic as well. I hardly ever notice my skipped heartbeats anymore. Why? "Is IR associated with arrhythmias or atrial fibrillation?" you might ask. You would be once again correct.

Atrial fibrillation, unfortunately, is associated with a much higher rate of stroke, cardiovascular disease, disability and death. Numerous epidemiological studies have linked atrial fibrillation with other obesity-related diseases such as hypertension and diabetes. Atrial fibrillation is strongly associated with IR and metabolic syndrome.[113]

There is mounting evidence that atrial fibrillation is not only associated with abnormal activity in the RAAS, but there is strong evidence that it is also related to the chronic inflammation produced by inflammatory adipocyte cytokines (in the belly fat).[114] Similar to its effect on skeletal muscle, we see a harmful effect on the heart muscle.

ATRIAL FIBRILLATION RISK

* Increased in insulin resistance
* Made worse with increased salt intake
* Decreased risk with coffee
* Worse when angiotensin system activated
* Increased with obesity

There is an increase in cardiomyocyte excitability with formation of fibrosis (scar tissue), enlargement of the heart, and fatty infiltration of the muscle. This all increases oxidative stress and damage to the heart. Studies show that aldosterone itself is associated with atrial fibrillation. Patients with primary aldosteronism have 12 times the rate of atrial fibrillation that normal people do.[115] Since intense aerobic activity, like marathoning or century cycling, provokes the RAAS, I recommend those with uncontrolled IR to avoid it.

Although this would not bother a non-insulin-resistant person like Faith, it could spell arrhythmia or disaster in someone with metabolic syndrome. That is another reason that light RT promoted in the Coffee Cure is probably the safest exercise for the typical insulin-resistant person trying to lose weight. I am not advising all people to avoid strenuous mountain climbing or marathon running. However, it is safer for the IR person to first reverse the condition before he chooses this intense an activity.

***

Your Skin on The Coffee Cure

Shortly after I began the three-year project of writing this book, I noticed a suspicious dark spot on my face near my right cheekbone. About the size of a penny, it progressively darkened over the summer.

I enjoyed writing while sitting by the pool, so I was getting lots of sun and its associated ultraviolet exposure. Despite the use of a hat, and sunscreen, it worsened. By winter, after my tan faded, the brown-colored spot stood out in sharp contrast to my pale face.

I resolved to make an appointment with my dermatologist, as the skin lesion appeared suspicious for a developing melanoma, a dangerous and often fatal type of skin cancer. I kept putting off the appointment as I never seemed to have enough spare time. When I rubbed my finger over the mole, I could feel its leathery texture, a bad sign. It was a solid color with sharp borders, a good sign. When I visited my family doctor, he was concerned. "Is it scaling?" he asked. "Yes," I quietly answered.

"See the dermatologist soon!" he commanded.

But being human, and much like my patients, I continued to procrastinate. Life got in the way. I spent less time outdoors. I drank more coffee, and it started to peel and flake. I scrubbed it and more skin came off. The leathery area also shrunk to the size of my little fingernail.

With the passage of six more months, it disappeared. As I write this, I find myself going back to the mirror to see if I can glimpse any trace of it. I cannot. I rub my finger over my cheekbone. Completely smooth.

Why? The studies on coffee are clear regarding both age spots and melanoma. Coffee is protective against both. Multiple studies around the world show that the more coffee one drinks, the lower the melanoma risk. The AARP study by Loftfield looked at 447,357 individuals who were cancer-free at baseline. 2,904 cases of malignant melanoma were identified over 10 ½ years of follow-up. Those who drank four or more cups of caffeinated-coffee per day enjoyed a 20% lower risk of melanoma.[116]

In Europe the results were more impressive. 500,000 patients were studied over 15 years. 2,712 melanomas were identified. In men, there was a 10% lower risk of melanoma for each 100 mls of caffeinated coffee per day. That translated to a 70% reduction in risk to those who drank 700 mls of coffee per day (around seven cups).[117] The researchers felt it was due to the caffeine in the coffee.

SKIN CONDITIONS & THE COFFEE CURE

Melanoma:
- Caffeinated Coffee can lower melanoma risk up to 70%

Basal Cell Cancer:
- Coffee can lower risk by 30%

UV Skin Damage:
- Coffee can reduce oxidative UV damage in a dose-dependent manner

Age Spots:

> • Coffee can be used topically as an extract to reduce wrinkles, age spots, and pigmented spots

Caffeine, administered either orally or topically, has a sunscreen-like effect. It blocks dimer formation of thymine molecules – a key step in UV radiation skin damage. Caffeine also induces apoptosis, pre-cancerous cell death. In human melanoma cells, caffeine helps to prevent melanoma growth, multiplication, and spread (metastasis).

Caffeine reduced the risk of other skin cancers too. Basal cell skin cancer was reduced by 10-30% with three cups per day of caffeinated coffee consumption.[118] Caffeine seemed to promote UV-damaged cell death, or apoptosis. Apoptosis is an important pathway for skin cells to block tumor transformation.

Finally, coffee can and does suppress simple age spot formation. Dr. Fukushimi studied coffee and age spots. Coffee and polyphenols were associated with a significant lower score of facial spots in Japanese women.[119] Dr. Cho in 2017 found that the chlorogenic acid in coffee reduced UV damage to skin cells.[120] He stated, "The results indicate that coffee's chlorogenic acid has the potential to be used as a preventative agent against premature skin aging induced by UV radiation."

There are dozens of other studies that employ coffee not only as an oral anti-aging skin agent but also as a topical one. Various coffee extracts have been used topically to slow wrinkling, spots, and signs of skin aging.

No discussion of the skin and the Coffee Cure would be complete without mentioning lactoferrin. Lactoferrin comprises about 1.5% of whey protein, so the standard daily dose of 60 grams of whey would give one about 1 gram of lactoferrin. This is skin friendly. It has been used to treat psoriasis, but it is most powerful against acne vulgaris. We know that whey lowers blood fats through triglyceride lowering. Lactoferrin also lowers the triglycerides contained in facial oils which translates into less acne. Lactoferrin can improve facial acne by about 30%.[121]

Given the Coffee Cure's powerful anti-inflammatory and anti-oxidative actions, it is clear to me that whatever my suspicious mole was, it was destroyed through apoptosis and by anti-oxidant defenses. Many small benign tumors develop every month in most people. Our natural defenses usually eliminate them before they can do us harm. (More on apoptosis, cancer and lactoferrin in Chapter 9).*

Individuals blessed with high levels of protective HDL may develop the start of artery plaques only to have them dissolve by their reverse-cholesterol transport system. Others may see cells initiate growth only to be killed through Apoptosis and anti-oxidant defenses.

It made perfect sense to me, as a physician, that if we focus more on getting our bodies maximally healthy, and consume diets rich in polyphenols, that we can stop disease in its tracks before it ever gets started. Meat and processed sugar both contain zero anti-oxidants. But here I was eating no meats or sugars, and drinking tons of polyphenol rich coffee, eating loads of phyto-chemical rich vegetables and drinking resveratrol-rich red wine.

If one polls a group of medical students and asks, "What cancer is the most prevalent?" you will hear many answers. But skin cancer is usually not one of them.

However, the fact remains that skin cancer has emerged as the greatest cancer epidemic of our time. There are more new cases of skin cancer each year than all other cancers put together. Melanoma, for example, was fairly uncommon in 1935, accounting for only a 1 in 1500 lifetime risk. Today, almost a century later, the risk has increased to 1 in 40.

---

*Although I procrastinated in getting my mole looked at by the Dermatologist; I DO NOT advise anyone else to do this. By all means, ALWAYS have a suspicious mole checked by your medical professional without delay. I was lucky. And I don't know what this discolored spot actually was. All I know now is that whatever it was, malignant or benign, it is now gone.

Your Colon on the Coffee Cure

As a medical student I spent one month working in the ICU of Ben Taub Hospital in Houston, Texas. My patient, a large grandfather, lay quietly in bed surrounded by beeping monitors. His hands were calloused, and he appeared fit. That had not prevented his heart attack, the reason for his stay.

Tubes invaded every orifice and the one that drained his dark urine would eventually kill him. I will call him "Big John." His family was the first that I had ever notified about a patient's death. About two days after his heart attack he began to perk up. He looked like he actually might make a full recovery; until he developed a fever.

I drew blood cultures and sent samples of his sputum and urine for culture. Sure enough, the tests came back positive for the growth of gram-negative bacteria. The bacteria were found throughout his bloodstream. Fecal contamination from his colon had infected his indwelling bladder catheter, and the organisms had then made their way into his blood circulation.

We started him on what were supposed to be lifesaving antibiotics. Only, they proved to be life-ending drugs. Within an hour of the antibiotic infusion, Big John crashed. His hands and feet turned cold, spotted, and purple while the alarm sounded. His blood pressure dropped to 50/0, dangerously low and incompatible with life.

Big John held on for a few hours while we pumped him full of dopamine, a drug that raises blood pressure. Bag after bag of saline fluid was pumped into his veins in an effort to save his life. His blood pressure briefly rose to 90. For a moment it looked as though we might save him. The senior resident who supervised me stood over my shoulder as he shook his head. "Gram negative sepsis is a bad condition. Sometimes the cure is worse than the disease."

Suddenly, Big John went into full cardiac arrest. We shocked his chest and gave him intracardiac epinephrine, but nothing worked. John was pronounced dead.

"Call the family," the resident commanded me. "It is time you learned how to do that."

"What do I say? That he died?" I asked.

"Of course not, tell them John took a turn for the worst and now you need them to get here right away."

"Okay," I stammered. I muttered to myself, "But what happened? We gave him the correct antibiotics, right? He was making a recovery from his heart attack."

The senior resident overheard me. "Endotoxin is what killed him. You see, Justus, when his bloodstream is filled with gram-negative bacteria and you suddenly kill them with loads of IV antibiotics, the bacteria break open as they die and release endotoxin. This endotoxin paralyzes blood vessel walls and it results in a massive drop in blood pressure. Nothing we know can reverse this. Not even dopamine. There was nothing you could have done differently."

Some 39 years later, scientists and physicians know much more about the leaky gut syndrome and endotoxin. Today, in 2019, we suspect that endotoxin also plays a major role in the development of metabolic syndrome and a host of related diseases, like leaky gut syndrome.

We now know that low levels of endotoxin otherwise known as lipopolysaccharide, or LPS for short, leak from the colon into our bloodstreams. This occurs much more in unhealthy people who eat high-fat or high sugar diets and who are sedentary. The intestinal walls normally are watertight and do not allow transfer of the bacteria into the bloodstream. However, in individuals with bad gut bacteria or those with leaky gut syndrome, LPS can leak through and can cause the release of inflammatory cytokines.

Many studies tend to show that metabolic syndrome is triggered by our Western diet which causes breakdown of intestinal integrity (otherwise known as increased intestinal permeability) causing bacterial endotoxin such as LPS to access our bloodstream.[122, 123]

It turns out that the Coffee Cure components can help neutralize this or at least slow it down even if we eat all the wrong food. If we look at Big John's condition, which is gram-negative sepsis due to endotoxin, chlorogenic acid has been shown to be lifesaving, not just helpful. In mice with gram-negative septic shock with the exact same condition of Big John's, the survival rate was less than 15% in a study.

However, in the same mice treated with chlorogenic acid, almost 90% survived. The coffee extract rescued the mice from the ravages of gram-negative bacterial endotoxin taking them from a 90% death rate to a 90% survival rate.[124]

Chlorogenic acid (CGA) is one of the main components of coffee. It reduces the damaging effects of the inflammatory cytokines in these mice by reducing levels of inflammation due to TNF-alpha in a dose-dependent manner. The endotoxin LPS elevated TNF in the septic mice. A tiny amount of CGA dropped the harmful inflammation by 40% while more dropped it over 80%.

Today's metabolic syndrome is caused by bad gut bacteria due to our high-fat and high sugar Western diet. This causes the leaky gut and the flow of LPS from the colon into the bloodstream. There it can cause endotoxemia (endotoxin in the blood) in an infected person like Big John or in the infected mice. However, in most cases of individuals with leaky gut syndrome, the levels are much lower and produce a long-term but low-level damage called chronic inflammation. This triggers the entire metabolic syndrome: elevations in blood sugar, blood pressure, triglycerides, and belly fat, etc.

We know that coffee and whey protein can reduce insulin resistance and now we know that it can also help reverse much of the leaky gut syndrome. It can also fight against the damaging effects of bacterial endotoxin, LPS. If that were not impressive enough, chlorogenic acid also helps seal up the intestinal wall preventing LPS from getting into the bloodstream in the first place.[125]

Whey protein decreases LPS intestinal injury by improving the mucosal barrier function, alleviating intestinal inflammation.[126]

The whey proteins themselves have been found to have numerous prebiotic effects on the leaky gut. For example: GMP, glycomacropeptide, a component of whey, supports growth of bifidobacteria, a good bacteria. The lactoferrin component of whey protein also supports two good gut bacteria; bifido bacteria and lactobacillus. Dr. Jennifer Causey, Ph.D., a research scientist, authored a treatise on the effect of whey on the intestines entitled, "The Whey to Intestinal Health".[127] She wrote that whey is strongly antibacterial and antiviral in its activity in the colon. It also enhances the immune system.

COLON DISEASE & THE COFFEE CURE

Increased Intestinal Permeability:

- Whey improves the mucosal barrier function
- Whey decreases LPS injury
- Lactoferrin in whey promotes growth of good bacteria: Lactobacillus and Bifidobacteria

C. Difficile Colitis

- Whey's IgG can help bind C. Difficile toxins.
- Whey is bactericidal

Whey increases the levels of immunoglobulins in the intestinal tract such as IgG, IgM, and IgA. This IgG has been shown to bind toxin produced by clostridium difficile, the organism responsible for the notorious C. difficile enterocolitis caused by excessive antibiotic use. Whey is one way to lower the levels of bad colonic bacteria without resorting to antibiotics. GMP has also been shown to inhibit the cholera toxin by binding to receptors in the intestinal tract.

Leaky gut, bad intestinal bacteria, and elevation of blood levels of LPS are all heavily researched today. In addition to the leaky gut initiating insulin resistance and increasing the risk for a whole host of leading causes of death like cancer, heart disease, stroke, Alzheimer's, and diabetes, it has also been implicated in many other inflammatory and autoimmune disorders including, but not limited to:

- Parkinsonism,
- Multiple sclerosis,
- Type I diabetes,
- Rheumatoid arthritis,
- Autism spectrum disorder,
- Inflammatory bowel disease,
- Crohn's disease,
- Ulcerative colitis,
- Irritable bowel syndrome,
- Celiac disease,
- Cirrhosis,
- Hepatic encephalopathy,
- Systemic lupus erythematosus (SLE),
- Uveitis. [128]

We have all heard about good bacteria and bad bacteria from the popular media. However, the message that we are getting that simply eating yogurt or acidophilus will cure your leaky gut is misleading.

Truly repairing your leaky gut requires reversing IR.

The components of the Coffee Cure have a powerful impact on the leaky gut syndrome and the pathology that we develop through our unhealthy dietary choices. The Coffee Cure components, whey protein and chlorogenic acid in coffee help the leaky gut. Once the LPS is in the blood, you can help neutralize some of the harmful effects, especially the effects of inflammation. RT has also improves colonic health. A sedentary lifestyle is associated with leaky gut and bad intestinal bacteria. TRE has been shown to reduce LPS-induced neural inflammation and memory impairment.[129, 130] Vegetarian diets are also associated with non-leaky guts and good intestinal bacteria.[131] While it is fine to consume yogurt and sour cream, don't forget the coffee and whey.

***

Your Mind on The Coffee Cure

"So, how many pounds is it today?" I asked my patient Penny.

Penny beamed as she answered, "Over 40 pounds Dr. Hope! I feel so good. Not just physically. I feel good mentally!"

"Wow," I smiled. "I am so happy for you."

"Dr. Hope, you may not realize it, but I have not been this thin in 25 years. I used to run and bike when I was younger. Now I am getting ready to join a gym.

"My mind is sharp. I remember things. I don't feel like I am in a fog anymore."

"Penny, I am sending you for some blood tests. In the past your triglycerides were over 500. I would bet they are closer to normal today. The studies show that triglycerides can actually pass through the blood-brain barrier and when they are too high can impair memory."[132]

"I will get my blood drawn on Monday," she said.

"How many cups of coffee a day do you drink?" I asked.

"Just like you said, I drink four cups a day, with 15 grams of whey protein in each cup."

"Perfect. Keep in mind that coffee is really going to help your memory even by itself. It is hard to believe, but coffee helps prevent age-related memory loss in most studies."[133]

When scientists poisoned rodents with memory-destroying drugs, coffee reversed the damage.[134] Coffee restores memory loss not only due to chemicals, but due to aging.[135] Coffee even helps restore memory due to drinking too much alcohol.[136] Caffeine by itself does not do the trick; it has to be coffee with all of its natural compounds. [137]

"Well, it has changed my life," she smiled. "I've been struggling with major depression these past 25 years. I put on almost 100 pounds due to those drugs, but I am determined to get off of them all. It has been so easy with your diet. My psychiatrist cannot believe it."

Penny's progress reflects how well the Coffee Cure diet affects the mind. Not only was she more mentally focused, she was much less depressed. Her depression relief did not come from the slew of antidepressant drugs that she had been taking the last 25 years, but from coffee, whey and weight loss.

Studies are clear that coffee improves depression. Some of this comes from Coffee's action on the Adenosine receptors. But some must also come from Coffee's effect on inflammation.

Believe it or not, according to the cytokine theory, most mental health disorders are related to inflammation.[138] These can range from depression to phobias to anxiety disorders. The higher the level of inflammation, the more resistant the depression is to treatment.[139] Inflammation has been linked to substance abuse disorder, generalized anxiety disorder, bipolar disorder, burnout, and anti-social personality.[140]

The problem is that the drugs Penny was given for depression also cause weight gain, which resulted in her developing the metabolic syndrome. She became so self-conscious about her overweight appearance that she did not want to be seen outdoors or in a gym, and stopped all of her exercise. In other words, the treatment for her depression made it worse.

The Coffee Cure program turned all of this around. Now she is so proud of her appearance that she is getting ready to join a gym. She is losing almost 10 pounds a month and has only six more months left to get down to her ideal body weight.

Anything that lowers inflammation can improve depression.[141] Studies using anti-inflammatory drugs have shown improvements in depression. The problem is that non-steroidal anti-inflammatories or NSAIDs can also cause harms such as GI bleeding and worsening of heart issues by raising blood pressure. However, coffee's chlorogenic acid is a powerful anti-inflammatory and can help not only with the weight loss, but it can also reduce inflammation while at the same time lowering blood pressure. It can also lower the risk for heart disease. NSAID drugs can cause disease while coffee reduces it.

PSYCHIATRIC DISORDERS & THE COFFEE CURE

Depression:

- Coffee blocks adenosine receptors and improves depression
- Coffee reduces inflammation which is associated with depression
- Coffee decreases suicide risk up to 45%

PTSD:

- Coffee reduces CRP
- Elevated CRP levels increase PTSD risk
- Whey at greater than 20 grams per day reduces CRP [greater than 3.0]

The CRP, a biomarker for inflammation, has been declared the villain in many inflammatory conditions. In fact, the higher the CRP, the greater the risk of death from cancer or heart disease.[142] Belly fat raises CRP. Coffee lowers it.

Coffee helps calm your mind by reducing depression, but what about PTSD? The Marine Resiliency study involved 26,000 war-zone deployed recruits. Military recruits who had higher CRP levels were more likely to develop PTSD.[143] After the recruits were deployed, went overseas, saw combat, and returned home, the resilient ones, the ones with low CRP, were protected against getting PTSD. By contrast the ones who had high baseline CRP got the condition. I believe that had they lowered their CRPs before deployment, by using weight loss and coffee, they would have become more resilient. They would have had less chance of contracting PTSD.

High CRP is at epidemic proportions in our country due to our inflammatory Western diet. Those with high levels of CRP tend to get all sorts of mental health disorders, not to mention physical problems. Angrier and more hostile individuals have higher CRP levels.[144] The higher the CRP, the lower the quality of life.[145,146]

MEDICAL CONDITIONS RELATED TO HIGH CRP LEVELS

- Cardiovascular disease
- Dementia
- Cancer
- Diabetes
- High blood pressure
- Obesity

CRP INSTIGATORS

- High-fat and high sugar diets ("The Western Diet")
- Insulin resistance
- Metabolic syndrome
- Diabetes
- Obesity
- High blood pressure
- Divorce
- Poverty
- Sedentary lifestyle
- Depression, bipolar disorder, PTSD, schizophrenia

What produces a high CRP you might ask? Getting metabolic syndrome or gaining too much weight. High blood pressure.[147] Divorce.[148] Having parents who divorce or separate before the age of 18.[149] Poverty.[150] Being the victim of a stalker.[151] Having parents incarcerated in prison.[152] Eating a high-fat or high-sugar diet.[153] High CRP levels are associated with poorer memory and greater disease as well as a poorer state of mind.[154]

What lowers CRP levels? All four pillars of the Coffee Cure. Four cups per day lowers it by 16.6%.[155] Weight loss lowers the CRP level. Whey protein (greater than 20 grams per day).[156]

Lactoferrin, the most magical part of whey protein, has a calming effect. It reduces stress-induced cortisol levels by lowering CRP.[157] Intermittent fasting lowers CRP.[158] What else lowers CRP?

Exercise and physical activity.[159] Prayer and meditation.[160] Tai Chi and Yoga.[161] Vegetarians have lower CRP levels.[162] If CRP is the devil to your mind, then the Coffee Cure Diet is the angel.

CRP REDUCERS

- Coffee consumption
- Whey consumption
- Weight loss
- Intermittent fasting
- Exercise
- Prayer
- Meditation
- Vegetarian diet

***

Your Lungs on the Coffee Cure

Parker winced as I injected his back. His muscles were in spasm. "How did the last month go for you?" I asked. "Well, aside from the back pain, I've been stressed over not working and not having any income. I just get depressed easily."

"Do you drink coffee?" I asked, knowing that coffee could help with depression.

"Yes. You know it helps my asthma big time."

"Really?" I asked.

"Yes, I don't even need my inhalers when I drink lots of coffee. It helps as much as my medication."

Parker's comment sent me back to the research. It turns out that caffeine in coffee is chemically similar to theophylline, the medication used in asthma inhalers. Technically, it is a xanthine, a compound found in plants that protects them against predators and microbes. Caffeine is xanthine, a methyl-xanthine to be precise. Theophylline actually has two caffeine molecules put together to form dimethyl xanthine. Both open up air passages and function as bronchodilators. Theophylline requires a prescription, coffee doesn't, although theophylline is a better bronchodilator. So Parker was correct. Coffee helps asthma.

A study measured respiratory function in coffee drinkers. Coffee drinking improved normal people's lung function by 3%.[163] This is kind of like the situation when normal vision is 20/20 but some people have super-vision and can see better than normal like 20/15. Only with coffee drinking, many had better than normal breathing function.

The 1983 Italian health survey found that the bronchial asthma prevalence was 23% lower in one cup per day coffee consumers, and 28% less in those who drank three cups per day.[164] Dr. Pagano felt that the beneficial effect on airways from coffee might not just decrease symptoms of asthma, but it might actually help prevent one from getting the disease in the first place.

Asthma is one thing, but what about COPD (chronic obstructive pulmonary disease)? Since cigarette advertising is legally banned in the United States, it is only the number four cause of death in this country. In Europe, India, and China, smoking is far more common. Worldwide COPD is quickly climbing to the number three cause of death behind only heart disease and cancer.

What effect, if any, does coffee and the Coffee Cure pillars have against this disease? Plenty. Much more than I realized before researching it. You may be surprised to learn that it is now increasingly thought of as an inflammatory disease, fueled by inflammatory cytokines of the same type produced by our belly fat. Cytokines like TNF alpha, and Interleukin 6.[165]

You may be surprised to learn that it is associated with insulin resistance.

In almost any inflammatory disease, the Coffee Cure pillars will tend to help. We need to start thinking about COPD like we think about knee osteoarthritis. Both diseases progress when inflammation levels are high. Smokers who have quit years earlier, still have ongoing active levels of inflammation in their damaged lungs.[166]

I think of my lungs as being like a house that I will need to protect me for the rest of my life. If my lungs catch an inflammatory fire, from say a decade of cigarette smoking, then after I stop smoking, that fire may continue to smolder. Imagine the house continuing to smolder as if there were active embers in the basement. As long as low-grade inflammation or smoldering continues, more tissue damage is taking place. More of your house gets destroyed with each passing day.

That is exactly the situation we see in many former smokers who have active COPD.

Dr. Leuzzi found that those COPD patients with the highest levels of inflammation were the most likely to die prematurely. Moreover, the higher the CRP level, the worse the lung function. A study in the United Kingdom analyzed the CRP levels in COPD patients. For every incremental increase in serum CRP, there was a corresponding decrease in FEV1 (the ability to force air out of the lungs in one second). There was also a corresponding reduction in FVC (the amount the lungs could inhale). In another study, Dr. Mann found that the higher the CRP level in those with COPD, the more quickly the lung function was lost.[167]

So how does one put out the smoldering fire of inflammation if one has COPD?

Dr. Sugawara found that by combining muscle strengthening exercises with whey protein supplementation, he could substantially decrease CRP, TNF-alpha, and Interleukin-6 levels. At the same time these patients also noticed improved breathing function and a better quality of life.[168]

Adding insulin resistance or diabetes to COPD makes the condition much worse.[169] It is like throwing a daily dose of jet fuel on those fires. Coffee, the first pillar of Coffee Cure, lowers the chance of getting diabetes and can substantially reduce insulin resistance. Furthermore, it lowers CRP levels.[170] We also know that TRE lowers inflammation.

What about obesity in COPD, you might ask? This is where the obesity paradox comes in. The problem for many COPD patients is actually too much weight loss. For years, the studies suggested that obese patients with COPD might outlive the leaner patients. But, as always, the devil is in the details.

It turns out that the more muscle COPD patients have, the better they survive. Sarcopenia, or loss of muscle, is extremely common in COPD. In particular, COPD patients tend to lose muscles in their legs, particularly the quadriceps, which are often 30% weaker than the rest of their muscles.[171] Dr. Polkey found that those COPD patients who weighed more with preserved muscle mass had better survival.

The more the insulin resistance, however, the more the muscle loss.

As you recall, a sarcopenic patient has a shortage of muscle and a surplus of fat even at a normal weight. This is similar to the situation in a COPD patient. They are plagued with increased inflammation and increased insulin resistance. If one could lose the fat but preserve or increase the muscle, one could improve a COPD patient's health.

Dr. McDonald and colleagues tested this and found it to be true. They designed an exercise program with weight loss involving resistive exercise and protein supplementation. They were successful in reducing obesity while improving their health. This was the first study of this kind in COPD.[172] It worked better than pulmonary rehabilitation, the traditional treatment. Those patients experienced less shortness of breath and improved ability to function and walk.

Specific exercises included biceps curls, shoulder presses, wall push-ups, squats, sit-ups, lunges, seated rows, and sit-to-stand exercises. Their diets contained 40% protein. The group lost 6% body weight, mainly fat, but they preserved their muscle mass. A study by Scott showed similar results.

The Coffee Cure pillars are similar in design to the McDonald program. The four pillars help the COPD patients lower inflammation and lower insulin resistance by increasing muscle mass.

What about other respiratory system problems and the Coffee Cure's effect?

Cystic fibrosis, for example, is a genetic disease characterized by abnormally-thick mucus causing inflammation, recurrent infections, and premature scarring of the lungs. Whey protein and its component lactoferrin, have been successfully used to help those with cystic fibrosis. Lactoferrin from whey has bactericidal activity against numerous strains of bacteria including E. coli, Salmonella, Shigella, Listeria, H. pylori, and Pseudomonas. Pseudomonas is a particularly nasty lung pathogen in both COPD and cystic fibrosis patients. Pressurized whey protein can lower the number of bacteria in pseudomonas lung infections.[173]

Lactoferrin has also been used as dry-powder aerosol in cystic fibrosis patients to provide antibacterial activity. [174] It has also been proven to be an effective weapon against Burkholderia, an opportunistic infection of the lungs in cystic fibrosis patients.[175]

Supplementation of pressurized whey protein in both cystic fibrosis children and adults decreased inflammatory markers such as CRP and IL8.[176]

Whey protein also improved levels of the antioxidant glutathione.[177] Whey has been shown to have strong anti-viral activity as well. It is effective against the common cold, influenza, and summer colds.[178] A controlled study showed that whey protein can actually help prevent the common cold.[179]

Dr. Vitetta and colleagues performed a placebo-controlled double-blind study to demonstrate this. They accepted 126 participants who reported frequent upper respiratory tract infections. 90 of them were enrolled in the study with 47 receiving the lactoferrin in blind fashion while the other 43 received only placebo for 90 days. The total number of colds during the study was 112 in the placebo group but only 48 in the whey-supplemented group.

I might point out that I also looked up Echinacea for comparison. Not to burst anyone's bubble, but the JAMA study in 2015 showed no association between Echinacea and cold prevention.[180] However, the lactoferrin component of whey has been shown to have a broad spectrum of antiviral activity through dozens of studies. Lactoferrin has antiviral activity against the RSV, the respiratory syncytial virus, the parainfluenza virus, the Asian influenza A virus, the Adeno virus, the ECHO virus, the Roto virus, and the herpes simplex virus.

The problem with prescribing antibiotics for patients with cold symptoms is that while antibiotics may help those with bacterial upper respiratory infections, they will not help someone with a viral upper respiratory infection. As I like to say, a viral cold treated with antibiotics lasts seven days and one untreated lasts one week.

The beauty of whey is that it is effective against both bacteria and viruses. The other problem with prescribing antibiotics multiple times for a person with recurrent respiratory infections is that it can result in the overgrowth of resistant strains of bacteria. The advantage of whey is that it does not produce such resistant strains. It can be taken daily; not only for its antioxidant effect or weight-loss benefits, but to help prevent all sorts of infections ranging from the common cold to upper respiratory infections.

Finally, there is evidence that whey actually enhances the body's natural immune defenses; it makes our own immune system stronger.[181] Whey acidic protein (WAP) can improve innate immunity and has played a role in HIV therapy.[182] Whey's lactoferrin, in addition to killing bacteria and viruses, is also a powerful anti-fungal and anti-parasitic agent. As I will discuss further in Chapter 9, it is also used to both prevent and treat cancer. What better reason to take it daily?

Whey, a strong pillar of the Coffee Cure Diet, plays a vital role in protecting the lungs from inflammatory, oxidative, and infectious damage. Coffee, the foundational pillar, a natural bronchodilator, is particularly helpful in those individuals with COPD and asthma. Dr. Alfaro found that coffee was associated with a lower risk of respiratory-related death and suggested that coffee consumption should be a "part of a healthy life-style leading to reduced respiratory morbidity."[183]

The Coffee Cure Diet is not just for weight loss. It can help you breathe easier.

LUNG DISEASE & THE COFFEE CURE

Asthma:

- Incidence of bronchial asthma up to 23 to 28 % less in coffee drinkers

COPD:

- Coffee lowers CRP by 16%
- Whey + RT improved COPD sarcopenia/shortness of breath/physical function
- COPD is associated with increased CRP

Cystic Fibrosis:

- Lactoferrin in whey is used as an aerosol to prevent Cystic Fibrosis-related infections

Respiratory Infections:

- Lactoferrin of whey can help prevent common cold
- Lactoferrin of whey has broad antiviral and antibacterial activity

Chapter 7
ALL DIETS ARE NOT CREATED EQUAL

"My weight has been a roller coaster, where I faithfully stayed on a program only to reach my goal, stop the diet, and balloon up bigger than I was before, or just lose interest and binge eat."

-Anonymous Dieter

Like many of my patients, Byron was a yo-yo dieter. He worked for years as a car mechanic, and his co-workers nicknamed him "Popeye" due to his impressive forearm development. All the turning, torqueing, and gripping of the tools had overdeveloped his "Popeye" muscles.

The burgers and fries from the fast food joint were located two blocks away from the garage where he worked, too convenient to resist. Byron was able to grab lunch and return to finish jobs between bites of fries and sips of his cola. The satisfying fats and fructose corn syrup caused weight gain. The extra calories were stored as fat, and Byron slowly became insulin-resistant.

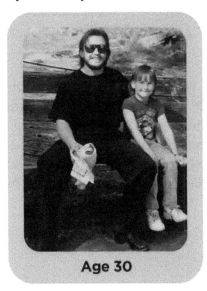

Age 30

Like Mandy, Byron became addicted to fast food and gained weight, but not immediately. After almost ten years of unhealthy eating, he began packing on the pounds. When Byron got up to 200 pounds, he went on a low carb diet. He ate burgers with no bun, drank diet coke, and ate no fries. He lost weight quickly, and soon he was down to 160 pounds. Much of the weight loss came from his muscles as the IR opposed fat burning. Proud of his 40 pound weight loss, Byron rewarded himself with some much-deserved carbohydrate.

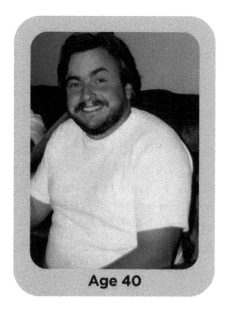

Age 40

Slowly, Byron lapsed back into his old eating habits, and his weight crept back to 200 pounds. Once again he repeated the process. Each time he lost 40 pounds on the low carb diet, 10 pounds of it was muscle. Each time he regained the weight, it was all fat. Progressively he lost more and more muscle. His once proud forearms shrank. People no longer called him "Popeye".

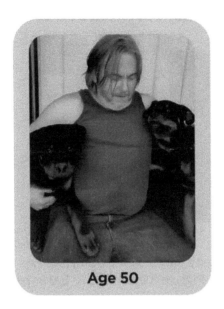

Age 50

One fateful day after a regain up to 200 pounds he received a call from his doctor. "Your blood sugar is 190! You are diabetic. You need to lose weight and fast."

Byron in fear for his life rapidly lost the weight. He starved and ate nothing but meat and fat. His weight plummeted to 150. His blood fats surged, and a major artery to his heart closed off. The unhealthy rapid weight loss had caused his heart attack.

Yo-yo dieting is the loss of fat and muscle with the regain of only fat. Over time this results in inflammation, IR, high blood sugar, heart disease, and in some cases cancer. It also results in the classic metabolic syndrome appearance of skinny arms, skinny legs, large belly, and the apple shape. Yo-yo dieting and metabolic syndrome can ultimately produce the unhealthiest form of weight loss, sarcopenia. Sarcopenia is defined as the muscle loss that occurs with disease or aging. It can be accelerated by yo-yo weight-loss cycles. Coffee can help prevent it.

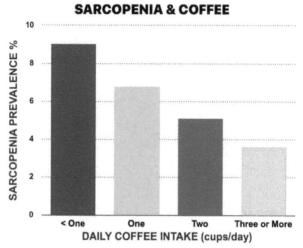

Adapted from Chung et al, Korean J Fam Med. 2017

Figure 29. Coffee & Sarcopenia

In many ways, Byron's dietary struggles mirror my own. When I decided to get healthy in 1997, it was because I had just spent five years going to night law school while working full time as a practicing physician during the day. I took care of patients with spine and brain injuries and found myself in court testifying about their conditions. The attorneys were always arguing about whose fault the injuries were and who had to pay for their treatment. I felt studying law would help me become a better doctor for my patients who seemed to end up in court.

However, those five years took a toll on my health. As anyone who works two jobs knows, there is no time for exercise. Drinking sugary sodas with caffeine and eating fast food on the road is inevitable. Eating dinner after 10:00 p.m. was also common for me. When I finally graduated, I had high blood pressure, high triglycerides, low HDL, and borderline blood sugar, all classic signs of IR. I had also gained in my waist. I knew that I needed to change my diet—and fast.

The problem was that I believed the government and medical establishment, that a low-fat diet high in carbohydrates was the healthiest solution. I also believed at the time that aerobic exercise would lead me back to fitness. I was wrong on both counts.

My new low-fat diet led me to increase my refined carbohydrates. I began eating rice, fettuccini and lots of bread. I even bought low-fat gimmicky products like rice cakes and low-fat foods. I ate high-protein bars, pretzels, etc. I switched to diet cola. I spent an hour each day on the elliptical trainer at the gym. I gave up all meats.

I did this for one year. At the end of the one year period, I didn't look healthier, and my waist had not shrunk. However, somehow I felt sure that I was healthier.

When I reviewed my laboratory studies, I was horrified. My cholesterol had risen 20 points, and my triglycerides had risen by over 100. I had given up meat, gone low-fat, and my numbers were much worse. Worse, I looked terrible. My skin was pasty. My chest had sunken. My once muscular arms had shriveled and appeared like thin sticks. My waist had expanded into a classic middle age spread at age 41.

I decided that I had to try something else. I had lost faith in the official recommendations like my patient Byron had. I went looking for answers, trying to find the best possible diet I could.

***

The Healthiest Diets on Earth

Some 21 years later, looking back now, I wish I knew then what I have since learned. A diet low in processed foods with little or no meat and high in dairy is healthy. Many of the longest-lived populations studied each engage in this type of diet.

The Greek Monks of Mount Saint Athos eat a diet mostly of plant-based carbohydrates that they grow in their monastery gardens. They eat no meat except for fish that they catch in the ocean about once a week. They eat fruits grown in their garden. They drink a glass of wine with dinner. They have two 36-hour religious fasts per week.

For generations this group of monks has been largely free of all major diseases like cancer and heart disease (with the exception of 11 cases of prostate cancer).

Clearly vegetables are healthy. Carbs contain four calories per gram making them low in energy density. You would need to be Houdini to get fat on vegetables. It's simple sugars found in refined flour and pastas devoid of fiber that surge insulin levels. Processing is the problem. As Jack LaLanne once said, "If it was not grown in the ground or once alive then don't eat it. Don't eat anything made by man." In short, avoid processed foods, vegetables or otherwise.

In the late 1950s a landmark study was begun by Dr. Ancel Keys and other scientists. They enrolled patients from nations including Italy, Greece, Finland, and the United States. They found that the heart attack rate of Finnish people was high while the heart attack rate of the people on the island of Crete in Greece was low, yet they both consumed roughly the same percentage of calories from fat.[184]

The fat in Mediterranean dishes from Greece came mainly from olive oil (a monounsaturated fat) while the fat from the Finnish group was similar to the U.S., mainly from meat and fried foods (saturated fats).

Like the Greek Monks of Mount Saint Athos, the most long-lived people tended to eat the least animal fats and consume the most unprocessed foods, like whole fruits, vegetables, and fish. They tended to eat the most olive oil, polyunsaturated fats, and the least saturated fats. They ate fewer fried foods, much less butter, and instead used olive oil on foods served cold or with bread.

Today, we know why Northern Europe and the United States residents lived an average of twelve years less than those who lived on the island of Crete. Studies show that olive oil lowers inflammation; it lowers amyloid plaque formation in Alzheimer's disease, and neuro-inflammation.[185] Canola oil does not.[186] Coconut oil does not.[187]

Fish oil is similar to olive oil in its beneficial effects.[188] It lowers inflammation and lowers the chance of getting neurodegenerative and heart disease. It is highly anti-inflammatory.[189]

Fried oils, on the other hand, are generally inflammatory and unhealthy.[190] Coconut oil when reheated can "pose a serious health hazard."[191] Saturated fats, like lard, when heated become so inflammatory that they actually chemically change into trans fats. Olive oil when cooked too long or for too high a temperature loses many of its benefits, but it is more resistant to heat damage than other oils.[192, 193]

If fish oil and olive oil are the best fats, then trans fats are simply the worst. Fish oil and olive oil consumption will help you live longer, and trans fats and saturated fats in general will shorten your life.

Trans fats produce the most obesity, cravings, and life-shortening effects.[194] Even fried vegetables like fried garbanzo beans known as falafel are unhealthy and fattening. They are similar to our US favored dish of fried potatoes known as French fries. Fried vegetables, far from being healthy, are the opposite.

You can buy fried anything, and it will be unhealthy.[195] Not only do deep-fried foods cause heart disease, they make you fat.[196] They cause a person with obese genes to crave them. They can even become addictive.[197] The more you eat, the more you want. Boiling, steaming, grilling, or simply eating food cold are much better alternatives for your health.

This brings us to the alpine paradox. Although the hypothesis that eating low to moderate dairy was "key" to the Mediterranean diet, the subsequent studies of the Swiss showed that although the Mediterranean diet was healthy, in general, the more dairy consumption, the longer the life.[198] All other things being equal, the Mediterranean diet is ideal for health and longevity with the caveat that more dairy is protective. The reason is the particular kind of protein found in dairy.

***

Whey is the Best Protein

Protein is a necessary ingredient in our daily diets. Proteins are made up of amino acids. There are some twenty different amino acids. Twelve of these can be manufactured by the body. The other eight are considered essential because they cannot be synthesized and must be supplied by the diet. Without this dietary intake, tissue growth, hormone production, and muscle function will be compromised. Protein contains four calories per gram, and it has almost a negative energy density as it takes so much metabolism simply to process it. High protein diets are associated with weight loss due to this thermic effect.

Proteins can come from both animal and plant sources. Animal sources include meats such as beef, chicken, and fish. Dairy contains whey and casein. Plant sources include soy, wheat, and nuts.

BIOLOGICAL VALUE [100 is perfect]:

- Beef 80
- Casein 76
- Eggs 94
- Milk 82
- Soy 61
- Wheat gluten 67
- Whey 92.

Animal protein from eggs, milk, fish, and poultry provide the highest quality ratings due to the completeness of the protein. Animal sources of protein have been criticized as somewhat less healthy due to the addition of saturated fat in meat and in the case of whole milk, saturated fat, and lactose or sugar. Whey protein with the fat and sugar removed from the milk is perhaps the healthiest. Casein is the other milk protein giving milk the white color.

Whey is from the clear liquid. Hoffman's study of 2004 looked at protein quality and found whey among the best due to its high concentrations of glutamine and leucine, both essential amino acids.[199] He felt that frequent ingestion of whey protein could improve health.

Protein up to 2.8 grams/kilogram was studied showing no prolonged ill effects. However, due to the theoretical issues with stress on the kidneys and calcium loss, I personally advise a prudent moderate and lower dose at no more than 0.5 grams/pound of body weight per day of whey protein supplementation which amounts to around 100 grams in a 200 pound adult or 50 grams per day in a 100 pound adult. This, in my opinion, allows the best of both worlds–complete animal protein benefit without the fat found in meat or sugar contained in milk.

So What Is the Best Diet?

What can we learn from all of this? Clearly, the world's best diets all involve low animal fats, sufficient protein, lots of unprocessed vegetables, and predominantly unsaturated fats. But even then, there are still a number of directions one can take from those. Let's end this chapter and this section of the book with a look at some of the ways my patients have interpreted the low-carb, vegetable-centric mandate, and how to shift them toward the healthiest version.

Low Carb: Pesco Style

My patient, Ron, proudly announced that he caught 10 large salmon on a recent fishing trip. "I have been eating smoked salmon, grilled salmon, and poached salmon. It is so good and it is so good for you," he grinned.

"I see your weight is up 18 pounds since last month," I replied. I observed him with his ruddy Irish complexion and noticed that he seemed to gain his weight in the middle. "Also, your blood pressure is up to 160/100."

"Oh, it always goes up when I am at the doctors," he explained. "It is fine when I am at home when I take it myself." The white coat syndrome strikes again.

"You know Ron, eating too much of anything other than plant food can cause weight gain. That can lead to metabolic syndrome, which you seem to have."

"I can take the weight off as fast as I put it on. You know my wife is Seventh-Day Adventist and she hates me eating any beef or even chicken. Fish is the only meat that she allows me to have."

"I know, I can relate. My wife is Adventist too. But here is the thing; if you have great genetics and gain your 18 pounds all over in your arms, legs, and hips, that is not going to hurt you. If you have IR like you and me where you put on any extra weight in the belly, that will shorten your life."[200]

"So, is salmon really bad for me?"

"Any meat, even fish, is nutrient dense. Salmon is one of the oiliest fishes known to man. If you eat too much of it, you will put on weight. So it is okay to eat salmon in a single portion with vegetables once a week, but not three times a day with multiple servings."

As I examined Ron's pained expression, I recalled this very issue. The studies show that too much fish will trigger IR just the same as regular saturated fat. At low intakes, less than 30% of calories, Omega III fats actually lower IR and do not cause weight gain. But in a high-fat diet where more than 37% of one's calories come from fat, even Omega III fat or extra fish intake *will produce* weight gain and IR![201]

A study of different groups of Seventh-Day Adventists revealed that those who ate dairy but no meat, not even fish, had 60% less metabolic syndrome than the Adventists that ate meat.[202] Then they compared the Lacto-ovo-vegetarian to the pesco-vegetarian Adventists. Pesco vegetarians are vegetarians with the exception of eating fish. Lacto-ovo vegetarians are vegetarians with the exception of eating dairy and eggs. The fish-eating vegetarians had only a 30% reduction in metabolic syndrome, and they developed it twice as frequently as Adventist-vegetarians who ate dairy and eggs.

It turns out that eating fish is not as healthy as we once thought. Too much fish creates visceral adiposity and is unhealthy. A study looked at Chinese who lived in Hong Kong with their traditional agricultural food intake.[203] Hong Kong has only recently been modernized and still is inhabited mostly by Chinese who were raised on farms. Singapore on the other hand is modern China, much more westernized with a high meat intake. Those in

Singapore have triple the rate of heart disease and metabolic syndrome compared to those in Hong Kong with more plant-based diets. Their difference was primarily their ratio of animal fats to plants fats. Those in Singapore had more than double the ratio.

My recommendation to Ron was, "Drink the coffee and whey before all meals. Begin RT, and limit your fish to one day a week for now." Fish is healthier than beef or poultry as it contains Omega III oil. It is good to consume fish so long as you don't eat so much as to gain weight. All weight gain for one who is at risk for metabolic syndrome is bad. However, if you want to avoid metabolic syndrome and its related diseases, it is best to gravitate towards an Adventist-style lacto-ovo-vegetarian diet.

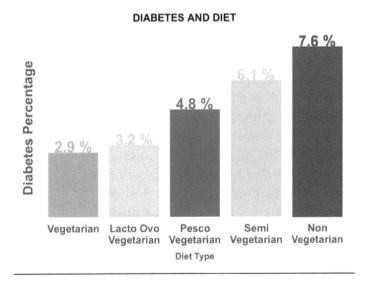

Adapted from Tonstad et.al. Diabetic Care. 2009

Figure 30. Diabetes Rate Depends Upon Diet

***

Low Carb: Meat Style

The moment I walked in to the room, I knew something was wrong. They say a good doctor has an intuition, a gut feeling, and can tell when someone is sick. Not just sick with the flu or cold, but sick deep down, sick in their organs.

"Shelly, have you lost weight?" I asked. She appeared sallow, her skin pasty. I had seen this color before in a patient who died of heart disease.

"Not really," she replied. "I have been camped out at the hospital. My mom was in the ICU after her stroke."

Shelly's blood pressure was 170/100. I knew that if she wasn't careful she would be heading down the same path as her mother. Shelly had classic salt-sensitive IR. Mine had started the same way. First, high blood pressure. Second, high triglycerides. Shelly's triglycerides had been so high, over 400, that she had been hospitalized three times for pancreatitis – a painful condition where one cannot stop vomiting. Basically, the pancreas clogs up with blood fats, the killer microns. Shelly was on strong pills to lower her cholesterol and lower her blood triglycerides.

She was on two medications to control her salt-sensitive high blood pressure. I knew that salt aggravated the condition and whey protein helped it. I had to ask her the obvious questions.

"Shelly, do you eat salt or salty foods?"

"Oh, not really, just a little Himalayan salt now and then."

Knowing that potassium could neutralize the salt damage I asked, "Do you eat enough potassium?"

"Oh sure, I take a potassium supplement each day."

"Not supplement, but natural foods rich in potassium, like avocados for example."

"God no, I hate those slimy green things."

"Well, how about mushrooms, do you like those? They have a lot of potassium."

"I ain't eating no fungus," she exclaimed.

"Do you like cheese?" I asked.

"Love it. So does my husband. He just lost 20 pounds on the Keto diet. He loves his steak and burgers too. He wants to lose another 30 pounds."

"It looks like you are down about 20 pounds since March. Are you doing the Keto diet too?" I asked.

"Pretty much. It works."

I noticed her arms and legs were getting smaller, but it was her color that really bothered me. She looked vaso-constricted. That is when blood vessels tighten up which elevates blood pressure. It is usually due to elevated levels of angiotensin II, which is a powerful vasoconstrictor. This is usually high in salt-sensitive insulin-resistant patients.

Over time (decades) the blood vessel walls get stiffer and thicker. The pulse wave velocity increases. The carotid artery, the main vessel leading to the brain, thickens. All of this dramatically increases the artery inflammation and oxidation, which skyrockets the risk of heart attack and stroke of the type in Shelly's mom.

I could sense Shelly, now age 55, was speeding towards the same fate as her mother. The studies are clear on meats and IR. They increase metabolic syndrome and the vicious cycle. The saturated fats in meats cause the liver to churn out more sugar through gluconeogenesis. Of course, this sugar is converted to free fatty acids almost as fast as it is made.

These fatty acids stimulate the Type I macrophages in fat cells to cause release of TNF-alpha and other inflammatory cytokines causing inflammation to the pancreas and arterial walls.

The saturated fats in the foods also stimulate the fat cells to release angiotensin II, constricting blood vessels and further driving up blood pressure. The angiotensin II in turn triggers the release of aldosterone, which causes water retention. The aldosterone itself damages the delicate insulin-producing beta cells of the pancreas.

SATURATED FAT (MEAT) PROCESSING IN INSULIN RESISTANCE

- Saturated fats (meats) digested and absorbed; converted to free fatty acids (FFA)
- Circulated back to liver; FFA stimulate IR liver to produce glucose (gluconeogenesis)
- Liver converts FFA to triglycerides, which are stored as belly fat (visceral adipose)
- Visceral fat attracts macrophages type I; immune response causes inflammation
- Inflammation triggers production of angiotensin, which is converted to angiotensin II by ACE (angiotensin-converting enzyme)
- Angiotensin II triggers blood pressure rise and aldosterone secretion
- Aldosterone increases inflammation and stimulates more insulin resistance

SATURATED FAT (CHEESE) PROCESSING IN INSULIN RESISTANCE

- Saturated fats (cheese) digested and absorbed; converted to free fatty acids (FFA)
- Circulated back to liver; FFA stimulate IR liver to produce glucose (gluconeogenesis)
- Liver converts FFA to triglycerides, which are stored as belly fat (visceral adipose)
- Visceral fat attracts macrophages type I; immune response causes inflammation which triggers production of angiotensin
- Whey in cheese blocks conversion of angiotensin to angiotensin II by ACE inhibition
- No blood pressure rise; instead a blood pressure fall
- No aldosterone secretion

- When dairy products like cheese are substituted for meat, the IR cycle is broken

If I could only talk Shelly into substituting dairy and eggs for the meat, we could help reverse this process. Dairy is rich in whey protein, which blocks both angiotensin II and aldosterone. It helps stop the vicious cycle of saturated fat begetting IR begetting aldosterone, which begets more IR.

***

Low Carb: Coffee Cure Keto Style

When the Atkins's diet first came out, I tried it and I loved it. I would go out to dinner at my favorite restaurant and order steak and lobster. As long as I avoided the mashed potatoes and bread, I was good. Down 10 pounds the first week, I felt triumphant. "What an easy way to take off weight," I thought.

My other favorite meal was the rotisserie chicken. Juicy and satisfying, it was pumped full of salt, sugar, and spices. I could polish off a few drumsticks for a quick dinner. It took a lot of soap and water to wash off all the grease, but I didn't worry at age 35 about its effect on my health. As long as I lost weight, I was good. Or so I thought.

As time wore on, a strange thing happened. My waist grew thick, and my arms and legs became weak and small. I got out of breath easily while walking or hiking. I didn't know about IR 30 years ago. No one did. [204]

Today metabolic syndrome has reached epidemic proportions not only in our country, but around the world. We also know from studies that high levels of fat and sodium promote further IR with worsening of the metabolic syndrome. We know that salt aggravates the salt-sensitive insulin-resistant patient's angiotensin and aldosterone system.

And we know that saturated fat can actually cause IR in normal individuals.

Today, I understand why my blood pressure increased with the high saturated fat, low carbohydrate diet. When something seems too good to be true, it probably is. While one can easily lose weight on a low carbohydrate, greasy-food diet, the price is increased IR and progression of the metabolic syndrome.

However, there is a way that one can still enjoy the benefits of the low carb approach without any of the drawbacks. I call it Coffee Cure Keto Style or "Lacto-Keto" for short. One eats low carb, but substitutes dairy, eggs, and fish for the greasy food. Fermented dairy products like cheese and yogurt are rich in whey proteins, which are associated with a lower risk of the metabolic syndrome. There is an inverse relationship between consumption of dairy and metabolic syndrome. That is, the more low-fat dairy that one consumes, the lower one's risk for metabolic syndrome and its associated diseases such as diabetes and heart disease.[205]

DAIRY & MORTALITY

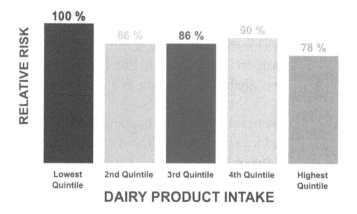

Adapted from Farvid et.al. Am J Epidemiol. 2017
Figure 31. Dairy Intake and Mortality

With the addition of coffee, whey protein, and time-restricted eating, one can utilize dairy in the Coffee Cure to lose weight rapidly with all the advantages of the Keto or low carb approach and none of the disadvantages. Simply substitute eggs, fish, and dairy for red meat and poultry. Liberally use cheese. Avoid whole milk due to its lactose or sugar content. I strive to keep all saturated fat, even cheese, below 10 or 15% of calories. A good goal is to keep all fat, saturated plus unsaturated, below 30%. Remember that above 37%, even unsaturated fat produces insulin resistance. I still enjoy my cheese and never have to ration it. Simply think of it as a garnish or condiment, and not as a main course.

If I had known about this 30 years ago, I would have employed it. The important thing is that we have good science today showing that the components of the Coffee Cure Keto-Style approach spins the vicious cycle of IR in the opposite direction. It takes advantage of the anti-diabetic, anti-inflammatory, and antioxidant effects of coffee's chlorogenic acid and the antihypertensive effects of whey protein and dairy to spin the IR cycle backwards.

***

Vegetarianism: Processed Food Style

By now you are probably familiar with the three types of vegetarianism: pesco, lacto-ovo, and pure vegetarianism without any animal flesh or products. However, you may not be familiar with the most popular form of vegetarianism—that is, the high carb processed food version. This is the type most practiced in the United States.

Just because one abstains from eating meat does not mean one need abstain from the pleasures of consuming frosted cereals and high fructose corn syrup or hydrogenated oils. Technically, vegetarians can even indulge in tasty fries, milkshakes, sodas, and all kinds of cookies, cakes, candies, and so-called "healthy energy bars."

This is the type of vegetarianism I tried in the late 1990s. After celebrating my law school graduation, I made a strict vow to myself that I would get healthy and cure my cholesterol and prediabetes problems without the need for lifelong medications. Vegetarianism seemed like the obvious choice.

The next week I was vacationing with my friend, Sid, and while he ordered pepperoni pizza at the local Pizza Hut, I made some vegetarian substitutions. Since they had no vegetarian pizza on the menu, and sandwiches were off-limits due to the lunch meat, I ordered two helpings of bread sticks.

"I can make this work," I thought to myself. While Sid ate eggs and bacon for breakfast, I had raisin bran cereal with milk and bananas. "A healthy choice," I thought. When Sid dined on steak, I barbequed veggie burgers. With monk-like discipline, I said no to meat and yes to everything else, be it the latest veggie burger, power bar, breakfast cereal, or processed food concoction. I actually began to enjoy processed food and sugar vegetarianism, my version of the lifestyle.

When friends would come to visit, I would offer them my favorite vegetarian dish, the half and half milk shake. I would use a half cup of sugar with a quart of half and half, add ice, and create the most delicious milk shake known to man. I then added an orange for health and flavor.

After a year of this type of vegetarianism, I retested my blood numbers. To my horror, when I rechecked the labs, they were not improved. My weight had risen to 210 pounds, my waistline had spread to 39 inches, and my triglycerides were up to 400. Moreover, my cholesterol on a diet of no meat whatsoever had risen to 210, the highest of my life.

Some two decades later with my wife, Faith, a devout Adventist, I was introduced to a healthier version of vegetarianism. It turns out that complex carbohydrates are an important ingredient to health, but high-fat cream, and simple sugars are a recipe for disaster.

The complex carbohydrates must be slow-digesting and contain natural fibers such as beans, avocados, and fruits. Faith never ate sugar or half and half, but instead relied on beans, brown rice, and vegetables, all of which were consumed in their natural form. This is considered a whole-food, plant-based diet. It does not include anything labeled low-fat or dietetic or anything that was not grown in the ground or once alive.

Rapidly absorbing sugar of the type found in all processed cereals drives up blood sugar, insulin levels, triglycerides, and plays havoc with one's health. It is also responsible for widening the waistline by aggravating IR. Although unprocessed meat with its cholesterol is harmful, it is much less so than consuming processed foods – be they meats or non-meats. Foods that are processed contain harmful preservatives and are often combined with chemicals, sugars, and trans fats.

True Adventist vegetarians stay away from meats, but they also avoid sugars and processed foods. They prefer eggs out of the shell, not out of a container. They stay away from gimmicks like low-fat, low sodium, or low calorie food that has been tampered with through the addition of sodium, preservatives, sugar, and/or chemicals designed to improve sales, but not health.

True lacto-ovo vegetarianism is the type practiced by most California Seventh-Day Adventists and the type that I recommend as part of the healthiest diet. Other types include strict vegetarianism with no animal products or flesh. This is simply known as vegetarianism. Because this lacks dairy products, which include whey protein, it does not block the angiotensin-aldosterone system to the extent that dairy-containing vegetarian diets do. Additionally, extremely low amounts of total fat intake, less than 6-7%, have been correlated with some conditions including a higher rate of hemorrhagic stroke. Adding low-fat dairy to a vegetarian diet is one way to obtain fat, but at the same time lower one's risk for cardiovascular disease.

Yes, all vegetarian diets are not created equal, and when people tell you they have tried the vegetarian diet and it did not work, simply ask, "What kind did you try?"

***

Vegetarianism: Adventist Style

Adventists are one of the most studied religious groups in the world. The original Adventist Health Study was begun in 1958 and is referred to as the Adventist Mortality Study.[206] It consisted of 22,940 Seventh-Day Adventists followed for five years.

The results were impressive. Adventist men lived an average of 6.2 years longer than non-Adventist men. Adventist women lived an average of 3.7 years longer than non-Adventist women.

Death rates due to cancer were 40% lower in men and 24% lower in women. Lung cancer was reduced by 79%. Colorectal cancer was reduced by 38%. Breast cancer was 15% lower and coronary disease was 34% lower in men and 2% lower in women.

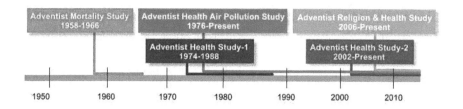

From AdventistHealthStudy.org
Figure 32. Adventist Health Studies

In 1986 Beason published a second study referred to as the Adventist Health Study-1 and looked at data from 34,192 California Seventh-Day Adventists.[207] In 1976 55.2% of this group fit in the category of Lacto-ovo-vegetarian, and there was virtually no consumption of alcohol, tobacco, or pork.

During the six-year follow-up in the Adventist Health Study-1, 20,702 medical chart were reviewed, and the results disclosed the development of 1,406 cancers with 2,716 deaths. A control group involved 112,726 non-Seventh-Day Adventists and was reviewed and the results were compared. Lacto-ovo vegetarianism was defined as meat from poultry or fish less than once a week and unlimited eggs, cheese, and dairy. Surprisingly, 22.3% of these California Adventists consumed between one and three cups of coffee per day, 4.7% consumed three or more cups per day, and 73% consumed less than one cup per day.

The results in Adventist Health Study-1 showed that the average Adventist male lived 7.3 years longer than the non-Adventist, and the average Adventist female lived an average of 4.4 years longer than other Californians. The reasons given in the author's opinion were the absence of smoking, the presence of a plant-based diet, the eating of nuts several days a week, and the maintenance of a normal body weight. The researchers felt that if the average Californian applied all of these principles, they could extend their life up to 10 years.

The principles also included reducing red and white meat consumption, more beans, and legumes. In the Adventist Health Study-2 which began in 2002, the goal was to accumulate 125,000 Adventists in the United States and Canada who would be followed for their health. Dr. Gary Fraser of the study found that there was an average of a 5 unit decreased body mass (BMI) between vegetarians and non-vegetarians which he felt was protective against type II diabetes. There was a significantly lower risk of metabolic syndrome.

Fraser wrote an article, "Ten years of life; is it a matter of choice?" [208] Fraser has published results that show Adventists who consume fruit three to seven days per week have a 70% lower risk of disease. Consuming fruit twice a day lowers the disease risk by 75%. Mills wrote that Adventist women as a group have the lowest risk of breast cancer compared to similar North American non-Adventists.

Meat consumption increased breast cancer risk. Mills also found that beans, lentils, and pears were protective against pancreatic cancer. Finally, Mills found that hormone replacement therapy, that is estrogen for women in the post-menopausal years, increased the risk of breast cancer some 69%.[209]

Hiryama studied a group of vegetarian Japanese with a lifestyle similar to Seventh-Day Adventists.[210] This Japanese group enjoyed one-fifth the rate of cancers of the mouth, pharynx, esophagus, and lungs and one-half the rate of stomach and liver cancer. They also enjoyed half the rate of cardiovascular disease. Giem found double the rate of dementia in meat eaters compared with most Adventists.[211] Phillips found three times the rate of coronary artery disease in Adventists who ate meat compared with Adventists who ate no meat.[212]

***

The Secret of Dairy: Fermentation:

It is difficult to feel satisfied without eating enough fat. The Mediterranean diet study showed us that eating animal fat (meat fat) except from fish was inflammatory, obesogenic, and life-shortening.[213, 214] The Greeks got most of their fat from olive oil or fish, both anti-inflammatory fats.

The Swiss, also long-lived, surprisingly got most of their fat from dairy: the so-called alpine paradox, and they also lived longer.[215] In spite of increased saturated fat consumption, the dairy fat not only was not associated with an increase in inflammation or obesity, but it was protective.[216] It was both anti-inflammatory and anti-obesogenic.

Many dozens of studies have confirmed this fact, but the best are the ATTICA and the Stancliffe studies.[217,218,219] Increased dairy fat like cheese, yogurt, and sour cream decreased inflammatory markers in the blood such as C-reactive protein, also known as CRP. Fermented dairy consumption was associated with lower blood pressures and more elastic arteries. Increased dairy, for some reason, had other factors that made it health promotive.

Fermented dairy includes cheeses that are acted upon by lactobacillus in similar fashion to yogurts, sour cream, and kefir. However, we are not referring to processed cheeses like Velveeta.

The studies show that pasteurized milk is not so healthy. The heating process removes/replaces many of the benefits of fermentation. I personally avoid it. When subtracting meat-fat like beef or poultry, I recommend that you add fermented dairy, olive oil, or fish oil to make up the difference. Dairy contains whey, and I personally believe this is a major reason that it reduces inflammation and blood pressure.

The secret of sourdough bread is the fact that it is a fermented product. Just as fermentation can transform dairy, it can also rejuvenate bread. Today with the epidemics of diabetes, obesity and inflammatory bowel disease, bread and gluten have taken center stage. But those who consumed the healthiest diets on earth did not suffer from gluten sensitivity. The researchers in the Seven Countries Study did not identify a need to create a "low gluten" bread.

This is probably because the food consumed in 1960 at the commencement of the Seven Countries Study bore little resemblance to the toxic creations so many consume today. The healthiest people in the Seven Countries Study, those residents of the isle of Crete, consumed bread produced through the traditional and ancient "Sourdough Fermentation" process. Their bread did not come out of a plastic bag. Instead it started with stone-ground wheat flour, which contained fiber. The dough fermented with the help of lactic acid bacteria for a full 12 to 24 hours, as the micro-organisms worked their magic.

The natural process involves breaking down the sugar, dissolving most of the gluten, and supercharging the dough with vitamins. The final product was an attractive baguette that was resistant to mold and possessed excellent consistency and taste. That traditional process of sourdough fermentation, once so common in Europe's Mediterranean countries, has now given way to our modern, Western and profit-centered abbreviated technique – the Baker's yeast method – that can be completed in just a few hours.

Consuming one slice of baker's yeast white bread is more like eating a candy bar with its high glycemic index of 71 and high fructose sugar content of 3 grams. It is also loaded with wheat gluten protein. By contrast, enjoying a slice of heavenly sourdough is closer to eating a high-fiber vegetable with its low glycemic index of 51, low sugar content of one gram, and absence of corn syrup.

The fermentation process can increase the amount of ACE-inhibiting enzyme, the ingredient so effective in reducing blood pressure in cheese. The lactic acid bacillus (LAB) confers antibacterial and antifungal protection to the sourdough bread, which lengthens its shelf life without the need to add the preservatives.

And I won't even begin to mention the bleaching agents, potassium bromate, azodiacarbonamide, and chlorine dioxide used to whiten the industrialized U.S. product. Of course, due to safety concerns, these have been banned in Europe.

So, you can understand why I choose sourdough-fermented bread whenever I eat it. Although most large companies don't take the time to do traditional fermentation, local mom and pop shops and even some mid-size companies are now selling it. But remember that even sourdough, in more than a few slices per day, may be too much.

***

A Word on Gluten

I once said, "We have had celiac disease and gluten for centuries. It would be crazy to think that suddenly everyone is allergic to gluten. It makes no sense."

But that was before I learned that insulin resistance has caused an epidemic of those individuals with breakdown of the gut barrier due to inflammation caused from our high- fat and high-sugar Western diet. Celiac disease, strictly defined as an auto-immune disease with intolerance to any gluten, and with positive antibody tests, is still rare at about 1/200 people.

However, up to 6% of the population, a growing number, have either a wheat-gluten allergy or hypersensitivity to gluten, termed non-celiac gluten sensitivity (or gluten-sensitive enteropathy), no doubt related to our Western diet.

Both the non-celiac and celiac bowel disease respond well to removal of gluten from the diet, often by using a rice-flour processed substitute made with toxic heavy metals. PubMed has published several articles demonstrating mercury and cadmium toxicity in patients consuming gluten-free diets.

However there is a better way. There is a non-toxic alternative. And it involves sourdough fermentation. No toxic metals. The sourdough fermentation process causes an enzyme, protease, to be produced. This enzyme greatly reduces the content of gluten, but prolonged fermentation can completely eliminate it.

If one is only sensitive, then regular sourdough bread may be a reasonable alternative, as it is naturally low in gluten due to enzymatic destruction during fermentation. I wouldn't self-diagnose, and as always, check with your doctor before you implement these dietary changes. Since I don't advise more than 3 slices of bread per day in one with active insulin resistance, and I advise against most pastas and cereals. This would constitute a low-gluten diet.

Gluten is not the main culprit in our current epidemic of bowel disease. It is really the insulin resistance caused by our Western diet and lifestyle that secondarily causes inflammation that breaks down our intestinal barrier. For the 10 or 15 percent of us prone to gluten allergy, we would never get it if this barrier remained intact. But today, many of us have gluten invading our immune systems through the leaky gut, causing the sensitive individuals to contract the disease. Once you have it, the only real remedy is to lower your gluten intake.

***

The Secret of Fermentation: Metabolism

Why is fermentation so healthy?

First, it has stood the test of time. The greek monks of Mt. St. Athos consume a fermented product, red wine, daily and they have virtually no recorded disease. The Seventh-Day Adventists consume cheese abundantly, and they live five to ten years longer than the rest of us.

Second, it is not a modern chemical process. Our experience with Crisco, margarine, trans fats, and high fructose corn syrup should have taught us by now to avoid eating anything "processed". It can't be good for you. No matter how attractive the packaging or wording. Low-fat or low gluten or low sodium likely means that somewhere along the line bromated or chlorinated chemicals were involved. It's never good.

Fermentation means metabolism by bacteria, and usually without oxygen. This process can occur in a jar, in a still, or even in a barrel. It is similar to when our bodies metabolize without oxygen, i.e., anaerobic metabolism. This is when lactic acid builds up in our muscles after intense exercise. However when bacteria ferment, often CO_2 gas is released causing the bread to rise. In the still, alcohol is produced from grapes as the sugar content falls.

In making cheese or yogurt, the level of lactic acid rises making the environment so acidic that all other organisms are eliminated – a very good thing. In bread, the gluten is softened and then destroyed. In Kimchi, the Korean equivalent of Sauerkraut, numerous anti-oxidants, anti-inflammatories, and anti-tumor agents are created, making it a superfood.

My favorite fermented food is Balsamic Vinegar, produced by bacterial breakdown of "must" consisting of the ground-up grape skins, stems and seeds. The must steeps in barrels fermenting for up to 12 years. The finished product is earthy, rich, and tangy as it has taken on the flavor of the grapes and the barrel.

I frequently enjoy a dish of fermented delicacies consisting of a main course of cracked sourdough bread dipped in olive oil, topped with mozzarella along with a salad of dark lettuce, tomatoes, and onions flavored with olive oil and aged balsamic vinegar, served with a good Merlot. Fermentation is the best way to improve foods.

FAVORITE FERMENTED FOODS:

- Sourdough Bread
- Rye Bread
- Sauerkraut
- Kimchi
- Kombucha Tea
- Sour Cream

* Yogurt
* Cheese
* Balsamic Vinegar
* Apple Cider Vinegar
  Red Wine
* Buttermilk Ranch Dressing

SECTION III:

FINE TUNING THE

COFFEE CURE

Chapter 8

COFFEE CURE TIPS & TACTICS

"This way to eat is so easy, everyone can be healthy with minimal effort." -D.M.

Over the years I have gotten to know every detail of the program inside and out as I have lived it. I have taken it to the office, on the road, on the plane, and on vacation. I have used it in restaurants, on the beach, on the slopes, and on the ice. I now reveal my closely guarded secrets that will break your plateau, keep you on track, and save you in your times of need.

The Cheat Day

"If you follow my advice I can help you," my personal trainer once told me. "But you know it is 90% diet. Any overweight person can come into the gym and throw around weights for two hours, but to be truly be fit you have to be disciplined in your eating. No sugars, sweets, or crap six days a week."

"What," I asked. "Six days?"

"Of course, you don't think I would deprive myself of my favorite foods all of the time do you?"

When you are just starting out on the Coffee Cure, the cheat day is perhaps the most important tip. One day a week, you can eat anything you want, as much as you want. If you eat perfect on the other six, you cannot hurt yourself (much). Your body simply cannot easily store the fat with empty liver glycogen.

I look back on that conversation with my trainer as a turning point in my life. There is good medical support for his advice. If you eat clean six days a week, your liver glycogen is low and empty going into your cheat day. Your body simply cannot store fat until it first replenishes the roughly 2000 calories of liver glycogen. However, if you cheat two to three days in a row, that is a different story. Once the liver glycogen is full and your body's energy bank account has been filled, your body is free to put in the extra calories anywhere it wishes, and it often chooses the stomach. That is why most people are not lean. If it were easy to achieve, many more would be thin.

My very first cheat day was like Christmas morning. I went out and bought all of my cheat foods. Mounds bars with chocolate and coconut, Reese's peanut butter cups, Hostess Twinkies, and of course M&M, both plain and peanut. I figured that I would indulge at noon, so in the morning I ate eggs and toast and went to the gym to do some cardio, my favorite, and some weights, my least favorite.

When I returned home, I popped in my favorite movie, Apollo 13, and laid out my feast in front of me. I unwrapped my Mounds and took a bite. I followed it with the Reese's and the Twinkies. For dessert, Rocky Road ice cream topped off the feast.

Later in the show when Apollo 13 informed Houston, "We have a problem" so did I. My problem was much lower tech. It involved frequent trips to the bathroom. When it looked like the astronauts might die upon re-entry, I felt the same. I couldn't watch the end because I was so sick.

Late Day Coffee

Learn the art of late day and after-dinner coffee drinking. While most of us are familiar with and enjoy morning coffee, most don't drink coffee in the afternoons or after dinner. Some connoisseurs may enjoy an occasional dessert coffee or espresso, but a sure fire way to succeed on the Coffee Cure is to make afternoon and evening coffee a daily ritual. Use decaffeinated unless regular coffee doesn't keep you awake.

You don't need whey protein late unless you have a craving for a snack. I simply enjoy it with a touch of cream. It helps my dinner settle by raising the incretin gut peptides that stabilize blood sugar. If I am taking a Friday afternoon flight, I enjoy it on the plane. If I am on the road, it keeps me alert. If I am at home, it simply helps me lose weight.

For the Coffee Cure newbie who may be experiencing a hankering for after-dinner sweets or popcorn, nothing works better than a cup of coffee and whey protein to kill one's craving.

Skipping Breakfast

"Wait a second," you may be asking. "Isn't breakfast good for your health, the most important meal of the day?" We have all been told this, but it turns out that it may not be true. The studies by Dr. Satchin Panda on time-restricted eating reveals that our Western high-fat and high-sugar diet does much more damage to our health when we have a shorter overnight fast. Cancer recurrence rates are much higher in those whose overnight fast is shorter than 13 hours compared to longer than 13 hours.[220, 221]

Since the 1970s, Americans have gone from a traditional three meals a day made at home to around-the-clock fast food and snacking up to five to six times a day. Many of us are led to believe that such constant snacking increases the metabolism. Certainly, eating once per day slows your metabolism. Ask any Sumo wrestler who employs this technique to gain weight. However, two to three meals a day seems to work fine for some of the healthiest people on the planet, such as Seventh-Day Adventists or the Mount Saint Athos Monks.

Skipping breakfast allows one to eat in an optimal circadian rhythm from 10:30 a.m. to 6:30 p.m. where the first meal "brunch" or "lunch" will likely be the largest. If you are like me, after a 16-hour fast you will be ravenous. That is when your digestive system is primed to handle killer micron surges or sugar shards most effectively. It is also after most of us have already enjoyed our morning coffee.

If you usually eat breakfast at 8:00 a.m. try my approach. Drink a cup of coffee with 25 grams of whey protein to suppress your appetite and delay breakfast until 10:00 a.m. Drink a second or third cup if you must, but wait until after 10:00 a.m. to eat. The food will taste better, you may eat more, and you will have less inflammation and lower insulin levels. By skipping breakfast, your eight-hour time window is moved forward. You will have dinner at 6:00-6:30 p.m. rather than 5:00 p.m. I don't know about you, but my worst temptations used to occur after dinner. By eating dinner late due to skipping breakfast, I am less tempted in the evening and can say no to the cheat snack.

Keep a Survival Kit with You At All Times

Keep your refrigerator stocked each week with a dozen hard-boiled eggs, half a dozen apples, four avocados, and a jar of Adam's peanut butter. It will get you through Phase II. Trust me. If you must go on the road, your survival kit will be modified. Apples, avocados, peanuts, almonds, and of course, whey powder. In the skies, skip the airplane food. It is poison. Break out your apple and nuts. Order some coffee and add some whey.

Cravings for sweets are greatest in Phase II. When you absolutely must have something sweet, indulge in my favorite: one sliced up apple with one heaping tablespoon of Adam's peanut butter. Use the Adam's as a dipping sauce for the apples. My rule is you may have a second tablespoon of creamy peanut butter only if you eat it with a second apple. This will not hurt your weight loss because of the high-fiber content in the apple – and after two apples and two tablespoons of peanut butter you should be filled to the gills with your sugar craving satisfied.

Boiled eggs are perfect for an extra snack or meal if you are hungry, and you will be. Studies show that when people substitute eggs for meat it reduces the incidence of metabolic syndrome. The eggs are one of your most potent weapons in Phase II.[222] Try to go two hours between snacks or meals. If I am too rushed to have brunch or am late for work, I simply grab an apple and an avocado. That is a full meal.

Your survival kit should always be stocked up in Coffee Cure Phase I with the four major food groups; eggs, apples, avocados, and a jar of Adam's peanut butter.

The Best Snack: Deviled Eggs, Coffee Cure Style

By week number five of the Coffee Cure, Byron was doing great.

"Well, I walked Frenchie into the ground yesterday," he said as he smiled.

"Really?"

"Yeah. He used to pull me and now I think I am exhausting him."

Byron had so much more energy, but he was starting to waver on the fasting.

"I am hungry all the time," he told me. "I eat, and I am hungry again two hours later."

"That is okay," I said. "That is normal. When you start building muscle, your muscles scream for you to feed them. One of my favorite snacks is deviled eggs, Coffee Cure style."

"How do you do that?" he asked.

"You boil up 18 eggs for the week and then chill them in the refrigerator. Pop the egg yolks out. Split the egg white into two halves. Squirt some mustard in it making it appear like a deviled egg. I like the sweet and hot mustard. Then have four to five halves with your coffee and whey protein. It is a great snack and is very filling. I do that whenever I am hungry between meals."

My faux "deviled" eggs got Byron through the hardest part of the Phase II. Try adding it to your survival pack. Another great snack is the chilled apple with a tablespoon of Adam's peanut butter as a dipping sauce. The rule is that you may have a second tablespoon of peanut butter, but only if you consume it with a second apple.

***

Monitoring Your Progress

Body weight is never going to be a truly accurate measure of health. The scale is a way to easily measure weight loss, but it won't tell you if it is healthy weight loss or not. Your appearance in the mirror will reflect if the loss came from muscle or from fat. If you can't trust the scales, then how do your monitor your progress? One answer is that you can get your body fat percentage measured. This is accurate. When your body fat lowers, you are making progress. However, measuring body fat may not be practical for most people. Simply look at your photos.

I studied Byron's photos at the beginning and after his third week on the program. His arms are noticeably fuller with triceps visible, while his neck is firmer with loss of the fat creases. His stomach is obviously flatter in just three weeks. One can measure their arms, neck, and waist. Measure your waist and hips at their widest dimension. Take pictures of yourself in the mirror, and then compare them each month. The scale will tell you if your weight is up or down. The photos and measurements will tell you if you have lost or gained fat or if you have lost or gained muscle.

Looking Under The Hood

Your numbers from your blood tests will also change as you get healthier and progress in your journey with the Coffee Cure. If you have good genes, you will already be one of those rare few who has a naturally high level of HDL and a naturally low level of triglycerides. However if you are like the vast majority of weight-loss patients, you will start with both numbers in the "bad" range. Your ratio of TG/HDL therefore can stand to improve and should get smaller as you lose weight.

This reflects that your insulin resistance is getting better. There is less sugar being diverted to the liver from resistant muscle, and therefore less sugar being converted to triglyceride, and less HDL is being used up to neutralize the triglyceride.

Take a look at the numbers of my patient Tonya. She started with a weight of 250. Her baseline Triglycerides were 450 and her baseline HDL was 35. Her ratio at the start of Phase I was 450/35 or 12.85. Six months later she was down 35 pounds and her triglycerides had dropped to 215. Her HDL was unchanged at 35, but her ratio had vastly improved to 6.1, a huge improvement in her health.

I advise you to keep track of not just your weight but those crucial longevity numbers. I get my blood tested every 6 months, however you may want to test yours more frequently as it is motivating to see the change!

Measure Your Strength

I can't tell you how many patients lose weight with just the first three pillars, but then forget to do the fourth, the strength training. They are obvious when they show up. Their arms are slender, and their grip strength is weak, yet they are down 35 or 40 pounds.

"So..." I ask as diplomatically as possible. "Are you doing the muscle contractions with your stretch bands or dumbbells 10 minutes a day?"

They first look at the ground. Then they look up. "But I have lost 35 pounds," they protest.

The New York Times Magazine reported in December of 2018 on a study showing that people who lifted weights even twice per week, for less than one hour total had a 50% reduced risk of heart attack and stroke compared with those who did nothing.[223] Doctors used to believe that one had to do cardio or aerobic exercise to gain a benefit to the heart. Not true.

WebMD reported in July 2019 on a study showing that men who could do 40 push-ups had a 96% lower risk of heart disease event compared to those who could do less than ten. Even those who could manage 11 or more push-ups had a 64% lower risk.[224]

The take-home message? Don't skip Pillar 4, the strength training. It could save your life, not to mention getting you better looking for the beach.

I get about an hour in total each week, usually over my three-day weekend, as I get too busy the rest of the week. The Coffee Cure doesn't preach 150 minutes a week of walking. Instead, we go by the science and advise at least an average of 10 or 15 minutes of strength training each day. These can be tiny 3 or 5 pound weights or simple stretch bands. Don't overthink it. Just do it.

And one more thing, the greater the grip strength, the lower the risk of death from all causes. Average grip is over 50 pounds for a woman and over 70 for a man. I strive personally for over 140 pounds. Faith's is 70 pounds. You can measure it on a Jamar Dynamometer, available at many physicians' offices.

***

Falling off the Wagon

In Phase IV of the Coffee Cure, falling off of the wagon usually means not being able to exercise. My patient Bill has been on the program now for four years. Before the program, his back always hurt and he couldn't sleep at night. He was never overweight and did not have metabolic syndrome; he chose the program to get healthy and fit.

"My back almost never hurts anymore so long as I go to the gym and keep my muscles strong," he says. "If I get called out of town for a family emergency or skip a few days, my back lets me know. Even if the pain is a level 9 or 10, I simply go back to the gym and half an hour later it starts to ease up."

Bill had been my patient for almost ten years after his back injury, and we had tried all kinds of treatments from pain medications to spinal injections to physical therapy. Surgery was even advised because his pain was so severe. But after he saw how the Coffee Cure helped me, he followed me to the gym and got a personal trainer. I advised him to do lots of light-weight repetitions up to 20 to 30 light pumps for each muscle group. Before this, he had already adapted to a semi-vegetarian diet.

He was in Phase IV before one year had passed. His office visits for back pain dropped from once every month to once every three months. He went off all of his pain medication. He put on fifteen pounds of solid muscle.

Then, while helping his parents fix their slippery moss covered roof, he slipped and fell, breaking his right hand. He had surgery with metal and screws. He was out of the gym for some two months, and his back pain returned.

"I can't stand it," he would say.

I advised him to do leg exercises like squats and lunges.

"No, I will just wait until I can get back to the gym."

He actually seemed to lose weight through losing muscle, and he was in danger of backsliding. Thankfully, three months later he was back to his modified-exercise program at the gym. His back pain disappeared.

For me, falling off the wagon means eating an extra mozzarella and tomato sandwich on sourdough bread or too many beans and cheese. Unlike Bill, I can actively gain weight and belly fat if I am not careful. When I overeat, I simply go with what works. I drink coffee after the meal to wash away the fullness feeling, and it works.

Studies show that drinking coffee boosts one's insulin secretion through gut peptides and slows the absorption of the food, keeping it in the intestines longer.[225] Both help reduce the chances that it will be stored as fat. Most importantly, it reduces that "stuffed" feeling. If I want to get rid of the feeling, I take an after-meal walk or do some after-meal resistance exercises. In combination with extra coffee, the exercise always takes the feeling away.

My muscle mass seems to do a good job of burning up any extra food that I consume. Muscle can be thought of as a fat-incinerating machine.

If I fall off the wagon with exercise rather than food, my approach is slightly different. Lack of exercise for three or four days leaves me with less energy. My arms start to soften, and I may notice some loose skin. I am 62-years-old, and my body is trying very hard to lose muscle. I usually don't wait for the scale to show me a rise in weight. I always go by the mirror first and the scale second.

If it is a weekend, then I do some catch-up. Two exercise sessions a day for two days and I am right as rain. It is sort of like making up a sleep debt. I call it an exercise debt and I try to repay it as soon as possible. The beauty is that a week off of exercise can be repaid with just four twenty minute sessions over two days.

For other diets, falling off the wagon means gaining 100 pounds back and then "rebooting" or basically starting over again. By contrast, the Coffee Cure is all about developing habits of coffee drinking, whey protein consumption, and daily RT. It involves eating your meals in an eight hour window, and saving cheat food for your cheat day. The cravings simply do not build up.

Once a person gets to Phase III or IV, they don't gain 100 pounds back, because they would have to unlearn four well-ingrained habits. With a typical diet, falling off the wagon would be easy as one simply giving up and going back to business as usual: all the wrong food.

With the Coffee Cure one would have to go against the 16-hour TRE, stop drinking coffee, eat cheat food everyday, and they still would not regain the weight because their well-developed muscles would prevent it.

The muscles, even if not exercised would still contribute to increased metabolism, calorie burning, and anti-inflammation through the myokine secretion and maintained mitochondrial concentration. This is what separates the Coffee Cure from a fad diet. It is a true lifestyle change. Once the four pillars have become well established, it would make one ill to try to unlearn them – just as in Bill or myself, we would get sick if we tried to change our eating habits.

Phase I, the beginning, is when a person might fall off the wagon due to a love of fast food, processed sugars, and an aversion to coffee, whey or fasting. But to get back on the wagon in Phase I, one simply needs to sip the coffee and whey and eat in the eight-hour window.

Don't worry at all about what you eat as a beginner. You could eat anything and you would still lose weight in Phase I. Even high fructose corn syrup containing snacks. Studies show that coffee attenuates fat storage even with high fructose corn syrup rich foods. The average person eats almost 30% fewer calories in a meal with a 40 gram whey protein preload.[226] In the PRISE study, even the whey group that did zero exercise still lost abdominal fat.[227]

With time-restricted eating, even when allowed to eat anything they wanted, pre-diabetic men consumed 20% fewer calories because of the eight-hour window.[228]

My advice to those in Phase I of the Coffee Cure Program is to simply put one foot in front of the other. You cannot help but succeed. Don't fear falling off of the wagon in the Coffee Cure.

***

Changing it Up: Meals

Phase II of the Coffee Cure is the easiest and where you will see the most weight loss. It is the phase where the art of RT is learned. The goal here is to adopt new habits; like drinking coffee at different times of the day, even after lunch. The second is adding whey protein to each cup. The third is consuming coffee and whey protein before each meal. This may involve switching to decaffeinated after 2:00 or 3:00 p.m. so one can drink coffee before each meal including dinner without insomnia. Finally, getting used to eating all of one's meals in an eight-hour time frame also takes a period of adjustment.

When one gets home from work late and plans a family dinner or meal out, one will usually skip breakfast to allow a 16 hour fast. If one, instead, prefers an early morning breakfast then the opposite may be true. An early dinner at 3:00-4:00 p.m. could be accomplished to allow a 16-hour fast before an early breakfast. Either way, one can get the daily 16-hour fast by postponing or skipping breakfast or instead by eating an early dinner. The TRE need only be done four or five days per week.

The weekends are free to eat any time you wish.

Give yourself four weeks to adjust to the changes in Phase II. For most, these will all be new habits to acquire and be made a part of your permanent lifelong routine. They are all abundantly healthy habits that reduce inflammation and oxidative stress. They also are powerfully anti-obesity, and your weight will fall even if you do not change your diet or begin any exercise. This is the beauty of Phase II.

None of my patients could say with a straight face that it was too difficult.

Simply sip coffee and whey protein drinks before each meal as if they were diet pills. Schedule your meals five days a week in an eight-hour time frame. This will produce some weight loss in almost everyone, but if you also restrict carbs and processed food intake, the average weight loss will be impressive resulting in around 8 to 12 pounds a month for most people.

This brings me to the topic of the ideal Phase II meal. Phase II is also when your IR is worse if you have typical Western induced obesity or IR syndrome like Byron, Mandy, and myself. Low carb or Keto style foods are best here with some modification. I would stay away from beef and sausage as they elevate the levels of free fatty acids in the blood which are known to aggravate IR. Avoid simple carbohydrates and high glycemic foods such as breads, pastas and rice while at the same time avoiding meat. Get your protein from whey and low-fat diary. I call this Coffee Cure Keto Style or Lacto-Keto for short.

As one progresses in the phases, Lacto-Keto gradually changes to Lacto-Mediterranean. Lacto-Keto means plant-based foods with carbs below 75 grams per day. Cheese and eggs are consumed in place of meat. Instead of adding unhealthy saturated fat calories, one adds calories from whey protein. No processed sugar. No sweetened yogurt or milk. No foods that will increase insulin resistance. Lacto-Keto means avoiding processed sweets or saturated non-dairy fats like pork, trans fats, and lunch meats.

Lacto-Mediterranean, by contrast, is where starchy carbs like legumes and potatoes are allowed, and carbs are increased up to 150 grams per day. We encourage Lacto-Keto in Phases I and II while progressing to Lacto-Mediterranean in Phases III and IV. Lacto-Mediterranean is where the restrictions on bread consumption are lifted provided one consumes only fermented products like sourdough and rye. More on Lacto-Mediterranean later.

My Phase II diet some fifteen years ago consisted of an egg and one slice of whole wheat toast for breakfast, chicken or tuna salad with vegetables for lunch, an apple and almonds for a snack, and vegetables with chicken or fish for dinner. That was with basic exercise. You can eat more times per day with more exercise.

For Byron, I advised something similar: an egg with or without one slice of toast for breakfast, an apple, peanuts, or almonds as a snack for lunch and salad with eggs and turkey bacon for dinner. Dressing is always with olive oil and vinegar. Balsamic vinegar is probably the best. I remind my patients to drink one-half cup of coffee with at least 15 grams of whey protein a half an hour before each meal or snack. If you get hungry, try my Coffee Cure deviled eggs as many as you want. They will not make you gain weight. Or have a portion of low salt peanuts with an apple as an alternative snack. They are both healthy and will not sabotage your weight loss.

For dinner in Phase II; I recommend a lean with green, meaning a green leafy vegetable salad with poultry or fish in a portion half the size of your fist. You can include tomatoes, fibrous vegetables, and dried cheese such as mozzarella or Swiss with an oil and vinegar dressing. Adding red wine is fine, keeping to less than two glasses for men and one glass for women. Contrary to popular belief, the wine will not raise your blood pressure, hurt your liver, or pack on calories if you stick to the doses mentioned.

It will help do precisely what is necessary in Phase II. It will help you reduce your IR and associated inflammatory cytokines, and it will turn down your livers gluconeogenesis (production of glucose). It will also load you up with anti-inflammatory polyphenols. In Phase II, you should never go hungry. If you find yourself starving, then by all means have some deviled eggs or an apple with peanuts. Remember to drink coffee and whey before the snacks. When one uses peanut butter, the type that I recommend with the apple should be Adam's peanut butter, the natural kind where the oil must be stirred in with the peanut butter.

If you must have beef or sausage, I understand. I once had those same cravings. Those cravings will be stronger in Phase II as IR is associated with leptin resistance and the hypothalamus is affected. It will cause you to crave sugar and fat and most likely beef and sausage. You may always indulge your cravings and eat your favorite cookies, cheese, chocolates, burgers, or fries on one day per week specifically on your cheat day within your two cheat meals. I would advise you to not indulge in any of the beef, sausage, or processed foods during the week because that will, unfortunately, sabotage your progress.

Remember, your body doesn't care what you do with two cheat meals a week so long as you eat clean the other six days. If you want more variety, all fibrous vegetables are okay and allowed in Phase II. All non-pork and all non-beef meats are okay. Simply stay away from pepperoni and processed meats which contain preservatives and/or nitrates.

All fish are okay in Phase II.

All dry cheeses are okay. Stay away from the gooey or processed cheeses. No Velveeta, cream cheese, brie cheese, or Havarti cheese. Cheddar, mozzarella, Swiss, and Parnassian cheeses are fine.

Use olive oil in cooking liberally. It is healthy and promotes anti-inflammation. I also encourage tuna fish with small amounts of mayonnaise and olives in your tuna salad. I would avoid relish until at least Phase II because of its sugar content. Haystacks made with turkey, salsa, cheese, lettuce, and tortilla shells are fine in Phase II as well. Stay away from vegetable oils that are solid at room temperature like coconut or palm oil. Be cautious and sparing with other vegetable oils like corn or safflower.

PHASE II: RECOMMENDED FOODS SUMMARY: LACTO-KETO

- All Cheeses, dryer cheeses better.
- All other dairy including cottage cheese, sour cream, yogurt (no sugar). No milk.
- Olive oil, balsamic vinegar, and apple cider vinegar
- All vegetables, especially fibrous like broccoli, carrots, cauliflower, brussels sprouts, kale
- Avoid starchy vegetables: peas, corn, beans, beets
- Mushrooms
- Meatless Monday
- Avoid red meat and cured meats like pepperoni, jerky, etc.
- Avoid pork and shellfish

- Keep carbs low; below 75 grams (Lacto-Keto). Limit bread to two slices per day. Use only fermented types like sourdough or rye.
- Natural nut butter ok (must have visible oil like Adams; No Skippy's)
- An apple a day as your main fruit. Avoid sweet fruits such as watermelon, pineapples or grapes
- Avoid figs, raisins. Avoid trail-mix. Nuts are ok.

Avoid starchy carbohydrates in Phase II; no beans, peas, beets, or corn. Celery, cucumbers, and tomatoes are fine. Radishes, cauliflower, brussels sprouts, broccoli, and leafy lettuce are fine. Steamed brussels sprouts with cheese are a favorite of mine. I like to take the added step of frying them in olive oil with some fried onions to give them more flavor before topping them with the melted cheddar.

Barbequed mushrooms with low sodium barbeque sauce and a small amount of ketchup served with lettuce, mayonnaise, and mozzarella cheese and one slice of toast are a favorite. Plank salmon barbequed with lemon and pepper are fine for all phases. They can be served with a side of steamed broccoli and cauliflower. All dinners can be enjoyed with red wine starting in Phase II. Remember the coffee and whey one-half hour before the meal.

An apple a day is a good rule of thumb. It is also loaded with antioxidants, polyphenols and it is low in glycemia. Even someone who is insulin-resistant must have carbohydrates to have reasonable amounts of energy. I do not recommend being in Ketosis for many reasons. Many studies have shown that Ketosis is associated with lower exercise performance especially in marathoners, athletes seeking to break records, and even in someone who is a couch potato.

I have noticed that Ketosis does not allow me to function at my best. Try taking a test while you are in ketosis, and you will see what I mean. The brain prefers glucose.

The apple is the best way to allow yourself some reasonable carbohydrates while staying out of ketosis and not aggravating the IR. I do not recommend macadamia nuts at least in Phase II or

Phase III. Walnuts are fine. Apple cider vinegar up to two teaspoons a day is great for health and you may use it as part of your salad dressing or enjoy it by itself. Sardines and crackers are a reasonable snack served with a non-processed low-fat potato chip such as a tortilla chip. One slice of toast a day is fine in Phase I, but I wouldn't increase it beyond that. Either enjoy it with breakfast with your egg or avocado or have it with your open-faced turkey sandwich at lunch.

Phase II is all about getting used to high doses of polyphenols with coffee and whey protein before every meal. It is also about learning to time your meals and suppress your appetite during the 16-hour fast. Many people are used to snacking in the evenings. I know, I used to do so. You don't have to totally give this up.

Certainly, you have three days a week that you can eat anytime you want, and those can be your nights for late-night snacking. During the four days, you will want to stick to the 16-hour fast as it produces lower levels of inflammatory markers. It raises PPAR-gamma. It is known to help reverse some of the effects of IR. Once you have mastered Phase II, you are ready for Phase III – the weight maintenance phase of the Coffee Cure.

Phase II is where Byron started with me. He had already lost thirty pounds, but had failed to lose visceral fat. His metabolism had stalled, and he was terribly unhealthy. He had out-of-control IR. He was experiencing chest pain daily. His blood sugar was out of control at 170, and he refused to take his medicine. He had resigned himself to an early death by also stopping his nitroglycerine and throwing caution to the wind. His waist when measure around the naval was 40 inches while his hips were 37 inches. The insulin resistance kept the fat in the abdomen. The goal for Byron and all others in Phase II is to lower insulin resistance with the four pillars which will cause a preferential loss of visceral fat. No other diet I know does this.

PHASE III: RECOMMENDED FOODS SUMMARY: LACTO-MEDITERRANEAN

- Same as Phase II except:
- Increase bread to two to three slices per day
- Add starchy carbs carefully: add peas, corn, and beans (Limit beans to every other day.)
- Increase carbs slowly to 100 to 125 grams per day
- Add Meatless Tuesdays and Thursdays

He overdosed on bacon fat and eggs while ignoring all conventional medical advice. He chugged coconut oil and guzzled Himalayan salt.

In Phase II, we turned Byron around by having him substitute turkey bacon for regular bacon and eat at least three times a day. We added an apple a day and we added a regimen of daily RT. In addition, Byron began drinking coffee and whey protein before each meal. The whey protein raised his metabolism. The RT also raised his metabolism and helped his starved muscles gather blood and glucose. He made remarkable progress in just 21 days.

Byron's weight dropped a good ten pounds. Blood sugar dropped approximately 55 points. His chest pain dropped by 90%, and there were visible changes in the mirror with loss of neck fat, loss of belly fat, and improved muscle mass.

Phase III meals are less limited because you have the hang of the program now. You are doing resistance exercises daily in Phase III and you have built some muscle and some metabolism from Phase II. Phase III is where you can eat a broader selection of foods. You will be less insulin-resistant in Phase III so your meals can change accordingly.

Phase III allows up to three slices of bread each day and allows the addition of more starchy vegetable carbs such as peas and vegetarian beans. I would reserve potatoes, rice, and noodles only for the cheat day. Phase III also involves the addition of a broader variety of fruits that might be a little higher in glycemic index such as oranges and tangerines. In Phase III I still recommend avoiding bananas, and pineapples.

Think of these sweet fruits as you would pastries. They are not ideal for those with IR as they spike both insulin and sugar shards. In Phase III you can consume more complex carbohydrates because you are exercising at least 20-30 minutes a day when most of these carbohydrates are now being absorbed into skeletal muscle.

A typical breakfast in Phase III will be two slices of sour dough toast with two eggs either fried or scrambled or omelette style. I often enjoy scraping off vegetable toppings from my cheat day pizza earlier in the week, heating them up, and topping them on the omelet or toast. Have fun with this. Use olive oil to fry up mushrooms, onions, vegetable pizza topping and use this to top your omelet.

For lunch have an open-face tuna sandwich with one slice of sour dough toast. Add one tablespoon of relish to your mayonnaise and olive tuna. Before lunch and all snacks don't forget your coffee and whey protein powder. Enjoy your apple and peanut butter in all phases.

One can actually enjoy selected fast foods in all phases of the Coffee Cure. In all phases one can enjoy Starbucks two-egg protein and bistro box minus the grapes, minus the biscuit, and minus the peanut butter. In Phase III one can have the peanut butter and the grapes, but still avoid the biscuit. For dinner out at a restaurant, one should be careful. At Applebee's or Outback, I would choose an Ahi tuna or a grilled chicken salad minus the grilled chicken. Simply substitute salmon for the chicken.

I find it is healthier than grilled chicken especially with the sodium content and portion sizes which are obesogenic. You can have your dressing on the side. Although, I prefer olive oil and vinegar in Phase III, you could even order Thousand Island or Ranch as long as it is served on the side and it is your cheat day.

I would avoid mixing the dressing into the salad as the portion sizes are way too large. Feel free to sprinkle peanuts in your salad if you are extra hungry. In general, avoid restaurant foods like the plague. They are fine for the cheat day with your family, but they are too high in sodium and hidden fats for daily fare.

With regard to the grilled chicken salads served in fast food hamburger restaurant drive-through, I would also avoid them. Usually they are served with high glycemic fruits like mandarins and contain high sodium, high-fat, and high sugar dressing loaded with condiments like croutons. Always de-crouton your salad whenever eating out.

Don't get me wrong, if it is your cheat day you can still order steak and lobster. I have ordered steak fajitas, my old friend, for years. Faith ate the beans and cheese while I devoured the steak fajitas. That is why the Coffee Cure works so well in the long term. You can eat whatever you wish at least on your cheat day every week.

In Phase III you will have now started to reverse much of the inflammation, and the IR, and some of the leptin resistance that caused your trouble in the first place. Your metabolism will be greater, and your body will be used to burning fat. By Phase III, your metabolic switch will be more flexible from the time-restricted eating. It will be used to turning off sugar burning and turning on fat burning.

Most importantly, your appetite tastes and cravings will start to change in Phase III, much like mine did. You may find yourself feeling a bit ill after the steak. You might notice that you don't sleep quite as well on a full stomach. You may decide that eating a hunk of animal fat is not as pleasant as it used to be.

That is exactly what we want.

When one avoids a certain food for a prolonged period of time and consumes it again, it is fair to say that they become more sensitive to its effects. If that particular food makes them feel ill in any way, they are more likely not to consume it again.

I learned as a college student the Sauce-Béarnaise syndrome is a term coined by Seligman and Hager. It refers to a story about a gentleman who dined on his favorite meat with his favorite sauce. Apparently he became quite ill that evening unrelated to the sauce or the food, and he vomited uncontrollably.

He then never ate Sauce-Béarnaise again, according to the story. There is a scientific basis for this.

If an animal eats something, and it makes them sick, they will stay away from it. I believe that is what happened to me. Whenever I ate steak after a long period without, it tended to overload my system with saturated fat making me feel rather ill.

In general, the less IR, the less leptin resistance, the more normal your appetite centers will work. This will also function to reduce your cravings, and if you are lucky your processed foods or meats will make you sick. Getting sick from the food is the best way to lose your cravings. It is fair to state that I have not had steak in the last three years. The beans and onions taste much better, and they never make me feel ill.

This brings us to the Phase IV meals. Phase IV is the portion of the Coffee Cure termed "polishing." It occurs generally after six to twelve months of Phase III, and it is where one has reached their target weight and began maintaining and developing a healthy base of muscle mitochondria.

PHASE IV: RECOMMENDED FOODS SUMMARY: LACTO-MEDITERRANEAN

- Same as Phase III except
- Keep carbs lower than 175 grams per day (i.e., .5 to .8 gram per pound per day)
- Increase bread to 4 to 6 slices per day
- Add Meatless Fridays

Phase IV is where the fine-tuning occurs. It is where one can eat almost anything without regaining any weight, but generally gravitates towards a modified Mediterranean or Adventist style diet. Mediterranean style diets are generally considered low in red meat and dairy, but high in polyunsaturated oils such as plant oils and olive oil. They are associated with low rates of diabetes or metabolic syndrome. They are also associated with longevity. In the traditional Mediterranean style diet one can consume fish.

The Greek monks of St. Athos consumed a modified-vegetarian style diet and they were remarkably healthy. The Seventh-Day

Adventist population has been extensively studied, and they consume a lacto-ovo-vegetarian diet. This is essentially a vegan diet with the exception of animal products from eggs and dairy such as cheese. By contrast, the Mediterranean diets include fish and some meats.

Seventh-Day Adventists have a very low incidence of diabetes and tend to live five to ten years longer than the average American principally due to a substantially lower risk of cardiovascular disease and a somewhat lower risk of cancer.

In Phase IV of the Coffee Cure, I recommend that you gravitate towards one of those styles. Since I live with a Seventh-Day Adventist, mine is decidedly more lacto-ovo-vegetarian but it incorporates many of the benefits of the Mediterranean diet including the addition of wine. Adopting such a lifestyle or diet does not mean that meat is never consumed.

It means that it is consumed at no more than one or two meals per week, the cheat meals mostly. My cheat meals almost never contain red meat or sausage. I also avoid most store-bought jerky. All-natural or homemade may be safest, or Trader Joe's brands without the nitrates. I incorporate all vegetables including corn, peas, beans (legumes), all nuts, and all fish. My diet includes the basics of the Coffee Cure; ongoing liberal use of coffee, whey protein, and time-restricted eating with moderate red wine intake.

I call my current diet Lacto-Mediterranean, and I am convinced it is healthier than either the Lacto-ovo-vegetarian or the Mediterranean alone. It is what I advise for all Phase IV graduates, and it is the pinnacle of the Coffee Cure. It consists of a standard Mediterranean diet modified to include moderate egg and cheese intake. It takes advantage of the Swiss Paradox, that those who consume a Mediterranean diet with more diary tend to live longer than those who consume less dairy.

Lacto-Mediterraneanism differs from the standard Adventist diet by including coffee and wine. The Coffee Cure four pillars can be viewed as training wheels that gradually adapt one to a complete Lacto-Mediterranean approach.

The philosophy is that one must change one's weight-loss approach depending upon one's degree of insulin resistance.

Beginners in the Coffee Cure with IR and waist larger than hips will need the Lacto-Keto diet to achieve Phase III where waist size shrinks to below hip size. Once a person with IR improves to that degree, they may add in more carbohydrate and the Lacto-Mediterranean diet.

The mistake that most people with IR make, and the one that I made, was adopting aerobic training with a Western diet which actually worsens IR although it may lower weight. Few can achieve Phase III with this approach, as the waist will not shrink as the persistent IR and related cytokines prevent it. I call this "myo-slacking" meaning lacking in muscle. Myoslackers may lose weight but they perpetuate IR through use of the wrong diet (Western fats and sugars) and wrong exercises (those lacking in RT).

With the ideal diet, Lacto-Mediterraneanism, I also encourage lots of activity such as walking, swimming, outdoor involvement, and fun with a core of daily RT to prevent muscle loss due to aging— the dreaded sarcopenia.

COMPARISON OF DIETS:

	Carbohydrates	Meats	Vegetables	*Dairy/Eggs
Standard Keto:	+	++++	++	++
Lacto-Keto	+	+	+++	+++
Mediterranean	++++	+	+++	+
Lacto- Mediterranean	+++	+	+++	+++

As one ages on the Coffee Cure program, one retains lean muscle mass while opposing fat storage. One uses all the nutritional and exercise strategies to oppose inflammation and oxidation. One maximally consumes polyphenols including red wine and coffee while avoiding the pro-inflammatory and pro-disease influences – no smoking – controlling and minimizing stress– avoiding pollution – and avoiding overconsumption of alcohol and – avoiding secondhand smoke.

One consistently supplements with Omega III, D3 and if indicated, the selective use of hormone replacement. In cases of low hormones, I would see a doctor. Low testosterone levels are also associated with IR and metabolic syndrome. Sometimes testosterone replacement may be indicated if one's level is below 300, or if the level of free testosterone is low.

One should avoid long stretches of sitting strategically by breaking up these episodes with RT. I was asked what one should do at the office. If one has a desk job like many of us or one has to commute with hours of sitting in a car, one can still bring stretch bands to the office, one can still stop and walk around in a rest area, and one can still alternate sitting and standing while studying paperwork. I would especially avoid the deadly duo of internet and television that has plagued our Western Society.

The easy way is to schedule your television and internet time at the end of each day after the sun has gone down. If you must use the internet as part of your office job, then alternate sitting and standing while at the computer. Perform exercise "snacks" with the bands. Studies show that if you don't sit longer than 15 minutes at a stretch, you can avoid many of the unfavorable health consequences of prolonged sitting.

Phase IV breakfasts for me include up to two eggs and two egg whites on toast or avocado toast. In Phase IV, three to four slices of toast can be consumed at breakfast depending on your metabolism, muscle mass, and physical activity. For others, Phase III or IV breakfasts could involve grapefruit, yogurt, or anything on our recommended Shopping Cart. Lunch typically includes apples, tangerines, grapes, cucumber sandwiches, tomato sandwiches, etc.

Crunchy sandwiches with Swiss cheese, open-face, and a tomato or avocado are satisfying and healthy. I like Caprese open-faced sandwiches made with basil and mozzarella. Vegetarian bean dip topped with cheese and served with Tostitos tortilla chips is fine. Frozen peas and carrots that are heated up and topped with mozzarella cheese are also healthy. I limit beans and bean dip to every other day to avoid triggering IR as these are high carb items.

Guacamole has become a frequent and favorite companion. Served with chips or vegetables for dipping. It can make a fine lunch or even an early dinner.

Learn to love your guacamole and always consider red wine with dinner if your doctor permits it. Haystacks are a favorite of Seventh-Day Adventists and are often served with or without grilled turkey. Essentially they involve tortilla shells with salsa, lettuce, tomatoes, cheese, and sour cream. The shopping cart in the appendix contains our typical grocery list. It is a good start for anyone entering Phase IV.

Look for our Coffee Cure Cookbook on Lacto-Mediterranean dishes soon.

In Phase IV the goal is to improve your progress by continuing RT, continuing time-restricted eating, and periodically check the scale and your photos. Monitor your waist circumference, arm circumference for signs of any increase in belly fat and if you notice these, dial back the carbohydrates to Phase III levels and increase the RT to six days a week. This should dial you back in very quickly.

The physician in me also recommends you keep very close tab of your blood pressure, fasting blood sugar, and triglycerides because these are sensitive markers of IR. The lower your IR, the smaller your waist. Simply visit your doctor and get laboratory studies every six to twelve months to make sure that you are continually dialed in. You will want your triglycerides below 150, your fasting blood sugar below 100, and your LDL cholesterol below 100 with the highest amount of HDL you can muster. You want your LDL to HDL ratio to be no higher than 2 to 2.5. Keep your hormones in the ideal range with your physician's help. Keep your TG/HDL ratio optimal, the lower the better, ideally less than 3.0.[229]

***

Changing it Up: Exercises

In Phase I of the Coffee Cure, it is all about drinking coffee and whey before meals as well as eating in an eight-hour time window.

Once you have that down then you can start considering exercise. If you already enjoy walking, cycling, or taking 10,000 steps a day that is fine. Those are not the kind of exercises that will reverse your IR. They may help in the short run, but in the long run RT is much more beneficial. If you are like Byron and enjoy walking your dog in the park, by all means continue. Just don't do that instead of the Coffee Cure exercises.

Do them in addition, not instead. Remember, I did one hour per day of Stairmaster with my heart rate at 140 to 150+ bpm. I did this for more than 15 or 20 years, all with no improvement in my Metabolic Syndrome, i.e., and no improvement in my Insulin Resistance. I used to be the ultimate myoslacker.

RT was what ultimately improved me.

An overweight individual with IR or metabolic syndrome is traveling away from their destination which is the state of health and leanness.

Imagine that you are driving away from your destination at 60 MPH. Before you can even begin thinking about getting to your destination you must slow down, stop, and reverse course. Before you can begin going in the right direction you must decelerate and stop everything you are doing wrong.

Turn off everything that causes inflammation. Stop smoking. Intensive aerobic exercise has been shown to worsen inflammatory markers in up to 40% of the cases. Although endurance exercises can create a temporary improvement in metabolism, the benefits are shorter term. Soon after stopping the aerobic exercise, one quickly detrains back to zero. This is not the case with RT.

Phase II is where I advise you to get to know your muscles again. Begin to remember the feeling as they get infused with blood and nutrients. In a typical metabolic syndrome or insulin-resistant patient, the muscles have been starved of both blood and nutrients for a very long time.

Begin by buying a pair of stretch bands and pumping them 10-20 times with each arm. See table 1. If you have just purchased this book and don't have the stretch bands and wish to start this minute then grab a one gallon jug of water. Stand or sit with your feet a shoulder width apart. Lower the full eight pound jug to your knees and then left it to your shoulders in a curling movement. Do this 10 to 20 times.

If it is too heavy or you feel pain, then stop and use half gallon or two-liter jugs. These weigh four pounds. Do this twice as many times up to 40. Now use the other arm and do another 20 contractions. Repeat each side twice for a total of three sets on the right and three sets on the left. Six sets of 20 contractions would be 120 repetitions or total muscle contractions. Congratulations, you have learned the secret of health. Muscles.

PHASE II: EXERCISE SUMMARY: BEGINNER

- Use stretch bands
- Use extremely light dumbells: 3, 5, or 8 pounds
- Use the KC-5 circuit: biceps curls, triceps pulldowns, band rows, chest flys, and walking lunges
- Do 5 sets of 20 repetitions the first month; 4 days per week
- Increase to 10 sets of 20 repetitions thereafter
- Other exercises as change-up: Modified "girl" push-ups, one-arm triceps extensions, planks, sit-ups, leg lifts, and sit-to-stands.

Muscle contractions burn fat and reduce inflammation. The better quality of your skeletal muscle, all other things being equal, the better quality of your heart muscle and visa-versa. If you have had IR for any length of time, the chances are that you have experienced skeletal muscle IR. This is unfortunately not only associated with a loss of fuel absorption and a loss of muscle strength, but is also associated with the muscles taking on unhealthy deposits of fat such as IMCL or intramyocellular lipids. This is also termed ectopic fat accumulation because fat does not belong in healthy muscle.

The more fat in the muscle, the worse it is for your health. Long standing IR like that found in type II diabetes or metabolic syndrome is also associated with increased pericardial fat, and you guessed it, with dysfunction of the heart itself. This dysfunction increases the risk of heart failure, arrhythmia, and even sudden death.

Cinderella for a Day

When one improves skeletal muscle insulin sensitivity, one also improves heart muscle insulin sensitivity.[230] As I like to put it, you are Cinderella for a day after a 20-30 minute session of RT. Your muscle will absorb glucose well. For the next 24 hours you will feel better, have more energy, and your blood sugar and insulin levels will decrease for at least 24 hours.

But to really get you moving in the right direction don't stop at six sets. Your goal is 20 sets of 20 reps per day by Phase III. Start by just doing ten sets daily of ten reps the first month of Phase I. Then increase to twenty sets of ten reps daily by the second month.

Remember it is not about lifting anything heavy. It is about contracting your muscles enough to get blood flow and nutrients in them. You can purchase your light stretch bands at most Big 5 Stores.

The easiest way to start Phase II is to buy a stretch band with handles. One can purchase these that allow anchoring in a closed door. While the stretch band is anchored in the closed door, one can easily accomplish the four types of exercise that I am recommending; elbow bends which are really bicep curls, as well as arm hugs which are really chest presses, as well as overhead band presses, and standing band rows which essentially involves a pulling movement toward the person.

In Phase III, I would use either heavier bands or heavier dumbbells perhaps by increasing five pounds. That means if one is using 10 pounds then one goes to 15 pounds. I recommend increasing the seated curls to five sets of 20 both right and left, supine press to five sets of 20 both right and left, triceps kickback to five sets of 15 right and left. One can also substitute a more aggressive exercise such as a triceps bench dip which essentially involves placing the hands behind the back using a bench to do dips.

PHASE III: EXERCISE SUMMARY: ADVANCED

- Increase to 20 sets of 20 repetitions; 4 days per week
- Add walking, yardwork, chopping wood, cleaning the garage, pruning hedges, or active household projects
- Keep television, computer, and social media "off" until sundown.

Finally, this might be the point where a full modified pushup can be changed to a full push-up if one feels strong enough and has no joint pain. Again, if one has any joint pain at all one should stop that particular exercise and check with their doctor, but continue all other body part RT.

This is a good time to remind you of the study that shows even 60 muscle contractions of RT improves Inhibitory Control, or IC for 24 hours. Those who did the RT session had more will power to say no to unhealthy food. It works. It worked for me. Let it work for your too.

In Phase IV you will have reached your ideal weight. You will be in maintenance, and you will want to polish your routine. Many of my patients in Phase IV have gone on to the gym and hired personal trainers, like my patient Bill, to do more high level work. This is certainly not necessary to do the Coffee Cure program, but it can complement it. A wider variety of exercises can be done with Nautilus equipment.

It is beneficial and can give you better control of inflammation and better improvement in your muscle IR. I recommend the addition of squats in Phase IV. The exercise ball is especially helpful for doing modified setups or wall slides, and I recommend leg lifts, sit-ups, crunches, and modified sit-ups with the Swiss ball. One can also work the back with dead lifts, although this should be done with some supervision to avoid back injuries.

Back extensions with the Swiss ball with proper medical clearance can help develop the hips. Seated nautilus equipment such as the abductor and adductor leg equipment is quite helpful as well as supine ham string presses. Exercises involving scissor kicks and hip kickbacks can help round out the program.

The TRX system is excellent as it uses the body weight for a variety of resistance exercise. I use it for rows. It can easily be adapted for home use, for those who don't like driving to the gym.

Kettlebells are perfect for very light weight deadlifts. These will improve posture and gluteal muscle tone. Always get a doctor's approval and some guidance before starting deadlifts as they are notorious for injuring the back.

Stretching can be done using Yoga or Pilates. I like Pilates as it helps strengthen and shape the core muscles. I recommend learning the "100". Get the book, "Pilates for Dummies."

The Coffee Cure does not require that you balance muscles, although one would seek to use a balanced approach anyway. However, to reduce inflammation in IR in this Coffee Cure program one can simply use the same exercises over and over as it doesn't matter which muscles you work, they will all tend to benefit your IR. The net result of RT is that all your muscles will absorb sugar and be healthier for it. Your goal in Phase IV should be perfecting the diet as well as perfecting the resistive exercises. You will want to get all of your muscles in the act. Not just the muscles most easily contracted. Phase IV is the time to acquire balance and symmetry.

When I am in a hurry to get to work, I can get 20 sets done in 20 minutes with my favorite music on a five-circuit routine. The goal is to complete all five sets before the song ends. Four circuits are 20 sets which are enough to satisfy my RT for the day, and I can accomplish it in 20 minutes. If you only have 5 minutes, then settle for the "Five and Fly." Anyone in Phase IV should be able to do the same thing.

There is no excuse for "lack of time".

PHASE IV: EXERCISE SUMMARY: EXPERT

- May decrease sessions to 3 days per week provided you are active and your waist is slim
- Take up a sport or join a gym
- Consider adding a personal trainer and balancing muscle groups
- Add a TRX system

One can try pulling exercises one day, pushing exercising the next; leg exercises the next, and abs the next. If you feel particularly energetic try pull-ups. If you are not at the gym find a low hanging tree branch. They even sell devices that can be placed in the door frame for pull-ups. They are a great exercise for back and lat muscles.

The goal in maintenance and polishing in Phases III and IV is 20 sets of 20 repetitions or 400 muscle contractions a day between four and six days a week. I would recommend older people (age 50+) limit this to four days a week with rest periods to allow proper muscle healing. For younger people six days a week should not be a problem.

Remember if you want to cycle, jog, or walk the dog, and you will because you will have extra energy as your muscles have been awakened, then by all means do so. But do so in addition, never instead of. There is a big reason the space program has cut out much of astronaut aerobic training and instead substituted strength training. It is because studies are clear on the enormous benefit that muscle exercise provides.

A study by Cavalcante in 2018 suggested that aerobic, but not resistance exercise could induce inflammatory pathways through TLR-2 and TLR-4.[231] He felt combined exercise, with both RT and ET was ideal because the resistance exercise could neutralize the inflammation caused by the (endurance) aerobic exercise. He stated, "Generally, combined exercise seems to be a good choice in most situations due to its positive effects on TLR expression and signaling." In other words, the possible inflammatory effects of aerobic exercise could be overcome through the anti-inflammatory impact of RT.

What Phase Am I In?

Whenever I see a patient in the Coffee Cure, I can usually tell where there are at a glance. I can see what phase they are in. Take my patient, Bill, my Phase IV superstar. He is age 50.

His waist is lean, and his shoulders are broad. He grips 150 pounds in the Jamar, and can do 53 pushups in two minutes. He appears a decade younger than his age and his numbers, blood pressure, blood sugar, TG/HDL ratio are all excellent.

Contrast this with Michael who is struggling with Phase II. His waist is larger than his hips, and both his blood pressure and blood sugars are a little elevated. His grip is 80 pounds. If he could take the last 20 pounds off his abdomen, both his blood sugar and blood pressure would fall as his belly-fat inflammation subsides. The instant his waist gets smaller than his hips marks the transition from Phase II to Phase III, from the weight-loss phase to the weight maintenance phase.

Phase III represents the greatest transition of the Coffee Cure. It marks the turning point in an IR person's health. For Don, my Phase III star, it marked where his waist shrunk smaller than his hips for the first time in decades. Down 42 pounds, Don is now squarely in maintenance where the goal is muscle strengthening, not weight loss.

His Jamar grip is 110 pounds and his pressure and sugar are both normal. However he is striving to raise his HDL by taking daily one hour walks and drinking a glass of red wine. He has also added heavier dumbbells to his strength training.

The obvious difference between Don and Bill is one of body fat percentage. Bill has well defined, well separated arm and legs muscles. His jawline is sharp and chiseled. Bill exudes energy and vitality when he enters the room.

Don is well on his way.

My advice for Don and many Phase III patients is to focus on RT because that is really the essential difference between III and IV. Bill accomplished his transition to Phase IV by joining a gym, hiring a trainer, and getting serious about muscle strengthening. The philosophy when hiring a trainer is to go high repetitions and moderate to low weights. Work on muscle symmetry and balance. Develop the chest and back equally. Develop your abs and hips equally. And don't neglect your legs.

You don't want to injure tendons or ligaments. Keeping the weight low will help prevent injury, especially in older people. In my opinion, the gym and trainer route is the easiest way to get to Phase IV, and this is good advice for Don to get to the next level.

On the other end of the spectrum, I am often asked what the main difference is between a Phase I and a Phase II client. The best answer, ironically, is similar to the difference between a Phase III and a Phase IV. The difference again is RT.

In early Phase I, the patient is consuming whey and coffee, the nutritional portion only of the Coffee Cure, without the RT. Once a Phase I has lost at least 10 pounds, and has added the full RT component, they are technically in Phase II.

The first half of the Coffee Cure is for beginners, the last half is for those serious about their health.

PHASES OF THE COFFEE CURE

PHASE I & II	WAIST	NUMBERS: BP & SUGAR	STRENGTH
• Beginner	* Larger than hips	* Poor Control	* Average or Low
PHASE III			
• Advanced	* Smaller than hips	* Good Control	* Good
PHASE IV			
• Advanced	* Smaller than hips	* Excellent Control	* Excellent

Chapter 9

DON'T DIE YOUNG

"Pre-malignant lesions may be present in a high proportion of healthy individuals, and whether these progress to an invasive metastatic fatal cancer can depend on an extraordinarily complex network. Insulin resistance and its associated hyperinsulinemia could form a significant strand in such a network."

—Dr. Ian F. Godsland

The preceding pages have clearly shown that the Coffee Cure will help you lose weight and live a better life. In this final chapter, we'll see how embracing the optimal diet and freeing yourself from obesity can help you live longer.

Abby's Diagnosis

Abby sat patiently as I walked into the exam room.

"Sorry I'm late," I said. "My last patient lost her dog and required extra time."

"Doctor, I don't know exactly how to say this. I've been your patient for 25 years, and I thought I would get to watch you retire one day. But I've just been diagnosed with pancreatic cancer. They say I have 3 or 4 months at most. I'm so sorry."

Abby was my sweet older patient; and when I say older, she was 10 years older than me. She was 71. Over the years I had experienced the privilege of also caring for her only son, Kenny. Kenny suffered a particularly severe case of the metabolic syndrome, and he had passed away suddenly from a heart attack in his thirties.

Abby withstood her grief over his death with grace. Her faith sustained her as she soldiered on through life. True to form, she now sat calmly and apologized to me for the terrible news that she had to bear.

Abby also had the metabolic syndrome, and although she was not 150 pounds overweight like her son, she still had insulin resistance. This had wrought it's damage slowly and now caused the development of cancer as the result of years of chronic inflammation and oxidation. Her 50 pounds of overweight was concentrated in her middle where it could do the most harm by creating a daily supply of cytokines.

The pancreatic cancer now would finish the job the insulin resistance had begun, and rob her of the last 10 years of her life. Why? What exactly causes cancer to develop in the first place?

Starving Cancer

That is, what causes our body's natural defenses to fail and thus stimulate cancer growth?

It turns out that sugar consumption, although highly correlated with heart disease, is not as clearly related to cancer.[232, 233]

There are good studies linking higher sugar consumption to higher risks of recurrence of colon cancer but science cannot simply claim, "sugar feeds cancer" because it doesn't. It is somewhat more complicated.

The studies are clear. We know that carcinogens like smoking, chemicals like PCBs, and ionizing radiation can do this. But by far the most common stimulant is obesity. Obesity fuels cancer cells through its chemical secretions, the inflammatory cytokines mentioned earlier. Body fat now has been classified as an endocrine organ capable of secreting various hormonally active substances.

Calle and colleagues looked at 900,000 adults in the U.S. between 1982 and 1998. They found an increased risk for cancer with obesity. The greater the obesity, the greater the risk.[234] Compared to those with a body mass of 25 or lower, the risk was 8% more for those 25 to 30, 18% more for those greater than 30 to 35, 32% higher for those greater than 35 to 40 and 62% higher with body mass greater than 40. For men the risk was 52% greater for body mass over 40.

The visceral or belly fat produces the most harmful chemicals. We know that insulin resistance, belly fat, and metabolic syndrome often occur together. Today, up to 40% of the U.S. population has one version or another of this deadly disease, in the past referred to as Syndrome X, or the Deadly Quartet. Although the belly fat produces its own harmful hormones, metabolic syndrome also drives up insulin levels. Insulin is considered an androgenic hormone, one that drives the growth of cancer – much like fertilizer grows plants.

Insulin can be thought of as the Miracle Grow that causes cancer cells to multiply and flourish. Even in non-obese individuals, high insulins levels are associated with higher levels of cancer mortality but when metabolic syndrome or obesity co-exist with excess insulin, we see large increases in cancer and cancer-related deaths.[235]

Tsujimoto and Kajio in 2017 studied 9,778 participants without diabetes or cancer. 6,718 were non obese.[236] Hyperinsulinemia or high Insulin levels were defined as greater than or equal to 10 micrograms/ml. The results were impressive. Cancer deaths were more than double in those patients with high insulin levels, even in those not obese.

INSULIN LEVEL VERSUS CANCER RISK

- Normal Weight and Normal Insulin Level =
  Normal Cancer Risk   = 1.0
- Normal Weight and High Insulin Level =
  Double Cancer Risk   = 2.0
- Obese Weight and High Insulin Level =
  Eight Times Cancer Risk   = 8.0

WAYS TO LOWER INSULIN LEVEL

- Lower Insulin Resistance
- Weight Loss
- Improve Blood Sugar Control if diabetic
- Improve Blood Pressure Control is hypertensive
- Intermittent Fasting
- Coffee Drinking

But if the person was obese and had high insulin levels, his risk of cancer was fully eight times higher than a normal lean individual. Clearly high insulin levels are a very bad thing not only in preventing weight loss, but very bad in terms of causing cancer.

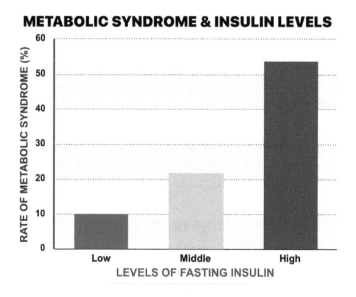

Adapted from Chen et.al. BMJ Open. 2018

Figure 33. Metabolic Syndrome and Insulin Level

The connection between insulin and cancer is clear from the studies. Trevisan and colleagues in 2001 found a 300% increase in colorectal cancer death in men as well as a 271% increase in women related to hyperinsulinemia.[237] Perseghin and colleagues in 2012 found an increase in overall cancer deaths by 62% in the one fifth of the group with the highest insulin levels.[238]

The insulin levels rise with obesity and metabolic syndrome as these both increase insulin resistance. As the body tries to make up for the fat-driven weakness of its insulin, it must make more of it, driving insulin levels up for every pound of fat gained. If insulin is the Miracle Grow of cancer, then blood sugar levels are the water that nourishes growth.

But sugar is where it gets complicated.

It's not the sugar one consumes in the diet. Instead, it's the average blood sugar level that waters the cancer. In a non-diabetic lean person or one with muscle, like Faith, blood sugar remains low while fasting and quickly returns to normal after eating.

In patients with higher fasting blood sugars, like those with metabolic syndrome and prediabetes, we see higher rates of cancer. The higher the fasting blood sugar, the more cancer and the deadlier the tumor.[239] Once the fasting blood sugar rises to diabetic levels, we see much more cancer risk.

Patients with diabetes are at much higher risk for developing cancers of the urinary track, liver, pancreas, colon, endometrium, and kidneys. A Korean study looked at 1.2 million diabetic subjects and found an increase in all cancers including a 24% increase in men and a 33% increase in women.[240]

We now know that in animal models, elevated blood sugar enhances spread or metastases of tumors. Tumors tend to grow larger in a high glucose environment even without excess insulin.[241]

Researchers feel that the inflammatory cytokines secreted from fat cells stimulate tumor growth. By now you should already know the cytokines by name: TNF-alpha and Interleukin-6. Knowing all this, what can we do to starve out cancer cells and prevent tumors from ever taking a hold on our bodies?

Caloric restriction studies show up to a 50% decreased rate of cancer.[242] Intermittent fasting studies show that 85% achieve a statistically significant weight loss. Even a single fasting interval (overnight) can reduce blood levels of glucose and insulin. If you are at high risk for cancer, then engage in time-restricted earing six days a week.

Killing Cancer

Apoptosis is the orchestrated and orderly destruction of defective cells. It is a natural process and vital to preventing cancer cell colonies from taking hold and multiplying. The more apoptosis, the less cancer, and the less apoptosis, the more cancer, all other things being equal.

Imagine your body uses a tiny vacuum cleaner to get rid of your decaying or damaged cells each day. As long as the vacuum does its job, you remain protected from mutant cells turning into cancer. But if your cleaner gets plugged up and stops working, you will have a problem. Abnormal cells will accumulate until they can do you harm.

The p53 gene, your body's natural vacuum cleaner, is responsible for apoptosis, the regular cleaning up and disposing of abnormal or old cells. It is known as the tumor-suppressing gene. Malfunction of this gene is responsible for the development of up to 50% of all cancers according to cancer researcher Dr. Ana Janic of the University of Melbourne.[243]

She further notes that the p53 gene is mutated in up to 70% of patients suffering from colon and pancreatic cancer. What if there were a way to boost p53 tumor suppressor function, a way to fix those broken vacuum cleaners or even enhance those not born with the best ones?

Lactoferrin, well-known to us as a component of whey protein does just that. It kills cancer by boosting our body's natural p53 function. Lactoferrin is being used against a variety of cancers as a form of natural, non-toxic chemotherapy. It is useful in treating brain, breast, colon, oral, head, neck, esophageal, skin, pancreatic, and bone cancer.

A remarkable study published in PLOS in 2018 showed exactly how effective lactoferrin can be against oral cancer. Cancer cell death or apoptosis was doubled in the lactoferrin group compared to control.[244] Cancer cell growth was reduced by 75% with lactoferrin. Lactoferrin not only will repair your broken vacuum, but will turbocharge those with mediocre models.

You may ask, "Why would my p53 vacuum stop working?"

Great question. The short answer is insulin resistance. The more insulin resistance, the less suction in your p53 vacuum. The long answer is inflammation and oxidation. They will ruin your vacuum. Cytokines, belly fat, smoking, and toxins all worsen p53.[245] Coffee, whey, muscle, and fasting all improve it.

Lactoferrin from whey is a proven weapon against cancer both before it forms and after it develops. It has broad activity against tumors, and this is not limited to its boost of p53. Oral lactoferrin suppresses tumor growth and helps other chemotherapies work better. It is now being tested to be used as an adjuvant to traditional chemotherapy in multiple cancers including breast, brain and pancreatic.

It helps patients who are receiving cancer treatment in other ways. It reduces the damage to the immune system that occurs with traditional toxic metal-based chemotherapies. It also reduces radiation damage from cancer-based radiation treatments. It helps reduce many of the unpleasant symptoms that occur with cancer treatment. Finally, it helps prevent the loss of taste and smell that often accompanies chemotherapy. Many of lactoferrin's benefits stem from the boosting effect it has on the immune system.

Lactoferrin hinders cancer by disrupting cell membranes, inducing apoptosis, and arresting the cancer cell cycle.

If you search PubMed with keywords lactoferrin and cancer, you will find about 800 studies. If you normalize your Insulin and blood sugar levels, you can imagine you are depriving cancer of much of its Miracle Grow and water supply. Consuming lactoferrin via whey protein can be thought of as adding a dose of Roundup.

What are some other ways to boost p53?

My favorite way to boost p53 aside from daily whey protein is to "train low". Training low refers to exercising in a carb-depleted state, a state where the body has consumed most of its glycogen. Numerous studies confirm that exercising while either carb or calorie depleted will raise p53 tumor suppressor function.[246, 247, 248] So I do my strength training at the tail-end of my overnight fast, just before I eat breakfast. For added benefit, during the workout, I chug lactoferrin-containing whey with my morning coffee.

Another favorite is to cycle my carbs down for one or two days each week. Following two days of carb depletion (75 grams of carbs or less per day) and the sixteen-hour fast, I do strength training for a double p53 boost. I shoot for this cycle at least once per week, and I advise my Phase IV high achievers to also do so, especially if they are at increased cancer risk for any reason, i.e., family history of cancer, personal history of cigarette smoking, diabetes, or insulin resistance. Take care not to over carb deplete; don't go more than two days as this can produce muscle loss.

Just two days before this book went to press, I encountered a brand new study linking TRE with cancer-risk suppression. It was too important not to include, so allow me to share it here. Dr. Monica Serra and colleagues published the Italian Study in Aging in June of 2019. They studied cancers that emerge during the aging process and found that TRE helped stop cancer from developing in older people. Although there have been many animal studies that suggest cancer suppression with time-restricted feeding, this was the first in humans. If you are aged or aging, and you don't wish to contract cancer, by all means eat only in an eight -hour window.

To summarize the effects of the Coffee Cure pillars on cancer, three out of four pillars either help kill or prevent cancer: Pillar 2, the lactoferrin from whey, Pillar 3, the RT, and Pillar 4, the TRE. And we already know that the remaining pillar, the most important one, coffee, Pillar 1, powerfully suppresses colon, liver, and skin cancers.

You would need to have a death wish not to want to use the Coffee Cure program.

***

Alcohol, Red Wine, Cancer and Insulin

"Regular and moderate consumption of red wine, perhaps one or two drinks a day with meals, should be encouraged. This would lead to a decreased risk of CVD (cardiovascular disease) as well as other conditions such as hypertension, peptic ulcer disease, respiratory infection, cholelithiasis (gallstones), nephrolithiasis (kidney stones), macular degeneration, Alzheimer's disease, and even cancer."

-Dr. Alfredo Cordova, The Lahey Clinic & Dr. Bauer Sumpio, Yale University School of Medicine

For years I feared alcohol as much as coffee, and for years I was wrong. Granted, the studies are clear that alcohol intake in general increases the risk for cancer. Approximately 3.6% of all cancers worldwide are spawned by excessive alcohol use-including liver, breast, and oral cancers.[249] However, as with coffee, the devil is in the details.

Moderate to low intake daily of red wine is the exception. Red wine at low levels has strong anti-cancer properties. Red wine represses both colony formation and spread of multiple lines of cancer in a dose dependent manner. It suppresses breast and esophageal cancer spread. Wallenborg noted red wine caused cell death in lung, colon, and cervical cancer lines.[250]

Red wine inhibited growth in oral squamous cell as well as human prostate carcinoma cells. Barron and Moore found that doses as low as .02% could suppress cancer colony formation. The most powerful wine the researchers found was Pinot Noir, the one with the highest phenolic component. The polyphenol compounds found in wine, especially resveratrol are thought to be responsible. Notably, Resveratrol by itself does not confer the same protection. Neither does white wine, even at ten times the concentration. It has to be red.

Red wine also raises Adiponectin levels by 10%.[251] Low levels of Adiponectin are associated with increased rates of most cancers. Higher levels are protective. Moderate red wine intake is associated with lower rates of many types of cancers. That is the major reason I choose to drink two glasses per day.

Red wine consumption has been shown to be protective against metabolic syndrome, largely due to the high polyphenol content of fruit-based wines.[252] Cherry wine has been shown to have even greater concentrates than grape-based.

Red wine has been extensively studied and is associated with marked reduction in almost every component of the metabolic syndrome. It lowers Insulin levels. It lowers IR, reduces waist circumference, and improves insulin sensitivity. It also turns off hepatic gluconeogenesis (liver production of sugar). It is associated with lower levels of inflammation TNF alpha. It tends to reverse the fluid retention, bloating, and sodium reabsorption caused by increased aldosterone secretion in those suffering from metabolic syndrome.

It has a thinning effect on the blood, which tends to counteract the blood clotting and prothrombotic effects of increased fibrinogen levels in metabolic syndrome. Wine is strongly associated with risk reductions of heart disease, arterial stiffness, and markers of atherosclerosis. RW reduces oxidized LDL levels, the most dangerous chylomicrons (killer microns), and it increases substantially the level of protective HDL. No wonder red wine and the Mediterranean diet are associated with so much reduction in the risk for metabolic syndrome.

There is a catch. More is not necessarily better. The sweet spot for disease reduction comes at two to three glasses a day for men and one glass per day for women. More than that is associated with an increased risk of breast cancer in women and more than two to three glasses increases the risk for liver disease such as cirrhosis in men.[253] Clearly, I do not advise people to take up red wine drinking if they are at risk for alcoholism. Still, compared to zero, three glasses a day of RW in a man can reduce his risk of metabolic syndrome by up to 50%.

The other catch is that all alcohol is not created equal. Although all alcohol in low doses tends to lower ones risk of cardiovascular disease, RW's health benefits are better. One study found a 33% risk reduction in heart disease for wine consumption, but only a 20% risk reduction with hard alcohol such as spirits like Vodka, Whiskey, and Tequila.[254] Clearly, hard alcohol just doesn't contain the antioxidants that rich red wine does. The risk reduction curve is J-shaped. None means higher risk than moderate consumption, but heavy drinking is much worse for health than no drinking.

Wine drinking doesn't just lower the risks for heart disease. It lowers the risk for getting most cancers through lowering Insulin levels and loading the body up on anti-oxidants.

Some studies do not suggest people start drinking wine to improve health, but other studies show that those in high-risk groups for heart disease might benefit. I would never advise anyone with a strong personal or family history of addiction or alcoholism to start drinking red wine, however. One can certainly get all the benefits of the Coffee Cure Program without it.

I would agree that those with metabolic syndrome tend to have the most to gain (no pun intended) and the least to lose by drinking red wine. Metabolic syndrome can triple ones risk of heart disease and premature death.

The red wine is one of the few tools that can raise protective levels of HDL and improve total to HDL ratios without drugs. It fights the bloat and water retention so typical of those suffering metabolic syndrome. Additionally, consumption of moderate red wine, contrary to popular belief, reduces blood pressure rather than raises it. Red wine also turns off sugar production in the liver by shutting the switch off for liver gluconeogenesis while at the same time increasing glycogen breakdown. This is actually a good thing because once liver glycogen is gone, fat burning is promoted. All alcohol is not created equal – but polyphenol rich fruit wine AKA red wine – Mediterranean style is protective against metabolic syndrome and many cancers.

***

Tex

When I read the studies of red wine, I am reminded of one of my first patients, Tex. He was a 60-something cowboy-type who had been drinking himself into an early grave. Tex had no family and when I rounded on him daily at the ward I couldn't help but feel sorry. Tex suffered from alcoholic liver disease.

Both of his eyes and skin were an orange/yellow shade. His belly was bloated to the size of a six-month pregnancy caused by fluid retention known as ascites. We had to restrict his dietary protein and fluids, but despite this his health was failing and he was not eligible for a liver transplant. Tex was dying and the hospitalization at the Veteran's Hospital was to ease his suffering. This would be Tex's last rodeo.

One morning when I came to visit, his bed was freshly made and empty. The chief resident told me that Tex had arrested the prior night. He had bled out internally when a blood vessel near his liver burst. Because I was his medical student, I was assigned to attend his autopsy.

I skipped lunch and showed up to the basement area of the Houston Veteran's Hospital. I entered the door marked "Pathology." The pathologist told me where to stand so as to not cause any interference with the procedure. He proceeded to take the scalpel and began opening Tex at the base of his throat down over his breast bone. He dissected out the heart and weighed it.

"Take a look at this vessel," he said.

"Is it the aorta?" I asked.

"Yes, and notice how clean it is. Absolutely not a speck of any cholesterol or plaque. Look here, the man has pristine vessel walls. The pulmonary artery is clean and the coronary arteries are widely opened."

"Why?" I asked.

He responded, "Alcoholics have clean blood vessels. The alcohol tends to cleanse their arteries. If it did not do so much damage to their livers it might actually be healthy."

Now that the pathologist had opened the abdomen, we examined Tex's liver. It looked like a large stone. "This is the problem," said the pathologist. "The liver is one big scar. The alcohol has destroyed it."

Studies are clear that in men two to three glasses of red wine or less per day does not cause damage to the liver. In women, one glass a day seems to be the limit.[255] The lesson is clear; to get the benefit of the alcohol-induced clean arteries and yet avoid the consequences to the liver, one must be extremely cautious about one's alcohol intake.

***

Fasting and Insulin

I use TRE (time-restricted eating) three to four days per week because of the way it makes me feel. It is like preparing for a blood test. If your last bite of food is at 8:00 p.m. and your first bite of food the next day is at noon, it allows you to fast for 16-hours. The closer the fast is to 15 or 16 hours the healthier.

Breakfast for me is 11:00 a.m. My last bite of food is often at 7:00 p.m. I sometimes drink coffee until 8:00 p.m. and then relax with a glass of wine afterwards. This gives me a 16-hour fast, and the effects are noticeable.

Going to bed on an empty stomach just feels good. There is no rock in my stomach from a hunk of animal fat, no GERD, no heartburn; just calm and peaceful sleep. I awaken the next morning fully rested.

However, when I see patients at the office, more than 50% of them are on antacids or anti-GERD medications. It is very difficult to talk them into giving up their meats or their nighttime eating habits. I used to share their heartburn pain, and I too took the occasional Prilosec or Tums. I never experience heartburn these days unless I have had a cheat meal the evening before, like chicken wings or pepperoni pizza. I wish all of them could experience the feeling of the Coffee Cure.

I can promise you no uncontrolled hunger on the Coffee Cure, but I cannot do it for you. As I tell my patients, "You are ultimately in control and responsible for your own health decisions and what you choose to eat matters just as much or more than any drug or medication you choose to take."

Fasting lowers insulin levels, but it is also associated with increased levels of insulin resistance, two apparently contradictory findings. Long fasts block the action of AS-160.[256] Strength training reverses this problem.[257] As long as one does not fast for too long, and regularly engages in RT, the fasting will lower insulin levels without increasing the IR. That's the beauty of TRE; it's long enough to help, but not so long as to produce adverse effects. The lowering of both insulin levels and IR is important due to the cancer and obesity promoting effects of high levels of Insulin.

INSULIN RESISTANCE VERSUS INSULIN LEVELS

- Insulin resistance produces a compensatory increase in insulin levels
- Fasting increases insulin resistance while lowering insulin levels
- Daily RT reverses this Increase
- Low carb and high-fat diets produce a short term lowering of insulin with a long term elevation of IR
- The four pillars of the Coffee Cure produce lower insulin levels and long term reduction in insulin resistance

The Night Shift

"You put on 10 pounds since I saw you two months ago," I told one of my patients with type II diabetes and metabolic syndrome. "And your blood sugar has jumped to 220. What has changed?"

"I got a new job. I work the graveyard from 11:00 p.m. to 7:00 a.m."

It turns out that nightshift work disrupts the natural circadian rhythm of sleeping at night and being awake during the day. This tends to disrupt a whole variety of hormonal patterns and cortisol secretion schedules that result in increased propensity for disease. Nightshift work according to a study by Sun in 2018 (meta-analysis of shift workers) is associated with a 23% higher risk of obesity and a 35% higher frequency of abdominal obesity.[258]

A study by Bescos in 2018 looked at healthy volunteers who were subjected to simulated nightshift work.[259] After only four days, they developed IR. The studies on time-restricted eating show that it works best when people do not go against circadian rhythms. Allowing a 16-hour daily fast is generally beneficial, but it is not so healthy if one must stay awake all night. I believe the optimal period for TRE fasting is one that coincides with our natural sleep rhythms. Studies show that it is healthiest to avoid eating any closer than four hours before bedtime.

Those who eat within two to three hours of the bedtime have higher rate of gastroesophageal reflux and esophageal cancer. If you must eat sooner to bedtime than four hours, a post dinner walk is suggested. Even a walk of 20-25 minutes following the meal will lower your chances of GERD and gastric cancer.[260]

So if you must eat within two to three hours of bedtime, take a walk afterwards. Some people eat their meals between 8:00 a.m. and 4:00 p.m. This is circadian-rhythm consistent and it is optimal for a 16-hour fast between the hours of 4:00 p.m. and 8:00 a.m.

The only problem that I notice with this is that many cannot go without snacking six or more hours until a 10:00 p.m. bedtime. I believe coffee and whey are vital tools to combat snack cravings following the evening meal. My patients tell me that in the evening, a cup of decaf with whey helps to give them more satiety allowing them to say no to the cookie or popcorn. I don't count the whey or coffee as breaking the fast.

The coffee does far more anti-inflammatory and anti-diabetic good than its miniscule effect on the fast. And the ACE inhibiting, glutamate-rich, and appetite-suppressing whey does much more good than its negligible effect on the fast. I drink coffee and whey an hour or two before I have my breakfast at 11:00 a.m. and it is a very pleasant way to gradually wake up and start the day.

***

All Fast Food is Not Equal

Fast foods are what got us into this fix. Americans wanted to save precious time and each time we used the drive-through and ordered a burger and fries, we did just that. We saved ourselves 15-20 minutes of meal prep time. Assuming three meals per day over the course of one week, we saved ourselves seven hours.

Over the course of a month, we saved more than one day of precious time that we could devote to something else like travel, going to the movies, watching television, or surfing the Internet. Over one year we saved ourselves two weeks. Over twenty years we saved ourselves a full year of time that we could devote to fun, family, and frivolity.

Then a cruel thing happened. We died ten years earlier of a heart attack, cancer, or we lost fifteen years from dementia. We actually lost the key thing we had expected to gain; our precious time. Nothing is worth your health.

The trans fats and energy-dense foods drove insulin resistance and metabolic syndrome. We all got a whopping dose of sugar shards and killer microns. Those lucky few with the good genes were able to whisk these away in their muscle sinks or with their protective HDL while those not so blessed, the majority, paid the price with belly fat, cytokines, inflammation and oxidation.

I like fast food as much as the next guy, but what if there were a way to get all the benefits of fast food without paying the price of disease?

In the Coffee Cure Diet, I have found just that. Starbucks has some healthy fast food selections if one is careful. Studies on fast food show that the more energy-dense, the more obesogenic; saturated fat like pork or beef, even high calorie cola, or extra sizes of fried potatoes all encourage metabolic syndrome. Anything in excess will promote weight gain, even fish. Like hard alcohol, it is too easy to slide down the slippery slope with concentrated fats and sugar consumption.

Trust me; you can't get fat on too many apples. I have tried it. You get a belly ache first.

You want low dense energy foods, often served cold, such as a Starbucks protein and egg bistro box. This contains half an apple, a serving of fresh grapes, and two hard-boiled eggs with a packet of peanut butter and a biscuit. I skip the biscuit and the peanut butter because it contains palm oil.

Bacon and sausage consumption are among the foods most highly correlated with metabolic syndrome. Cereal, white bread, and jams are also highly correlated. Way down lower are dried cheeses and eggs which are not only not correlated but inversely correlated. In general, moderate egg consumption is associated with a reduced risk of metabolic syndrome.

FOODS ASSOCIATED WITH INSULIN RESISTANCE

- Bacon
- Sausage
- Cereal
- White Bread
- Jam

Starbucks spinach and egg feta wraps are equally good choices to help lower metabolic syndrome risks. The egg Gouda sandwich minus the bacon is also favorable.

FOODS ASSOCIATED WITH INSULIN SENSITIVITY

- Cheese
- Eggs (Less than 7 per week)
- Fish
- Vegetables
- Coffee
- Whey Containing

Fast food doesn't have to increase your risk for metabolic syndrome. Choose fruit and vegetable selections and egg and cheese choices, avoid sugary sodas, fatty fries, beef, and pork, and avoid high sodium items.

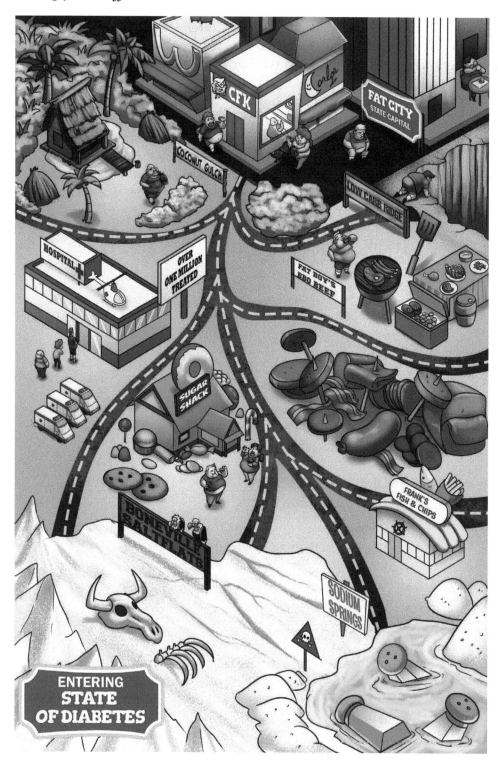

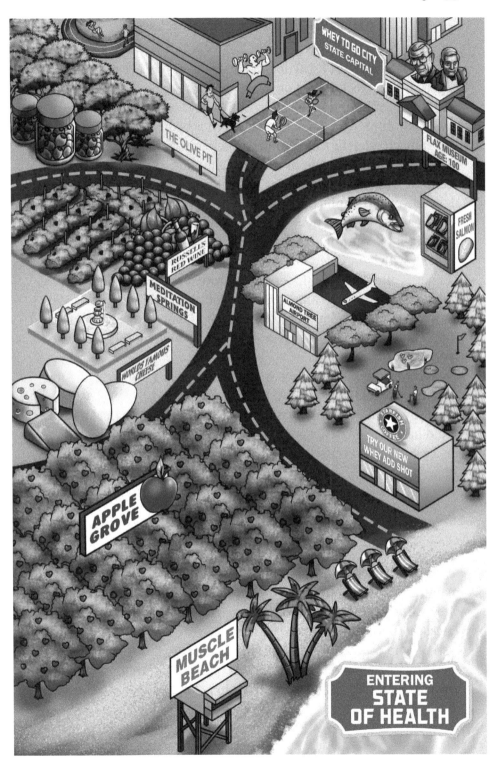

Healthy Fast Food: Starbucks Style

As a busy doctor, I still do not have time to prepare my own food especially on workdays. For some five years now I have enjoyed Starbucks coffee and meals at least five days each week, 52 weeks a year, year after year. They know my order by heart. Grande coffee, two spinach egg feta wraps, and a protein bistro-box. After my apple and tangerine from home and a jar of almonds, as well as my special blend of whey protein and my KC creamer, you have my average daily meal plan minus breakfast.

Breakfast which I have at home is either two or three eggs and two slices of sourdough toast or two slices of toast with avocado topped with sun-dried tomatoes and nutritional yeast powder. Dinner is often the remainder of my protein bistro-box on the drive home plus an apple or almonds, plus coffee and KC, of course. Why does this work? It is low in saturated fat and dairy and eggs are fairly safe. There are no trans-fats so typical of the fast food burger and fry establishment.

I enjoy the convenience of fast food, but I try to avoid the negative effects to my health. I find it ironic that Byron developed his IR by dining on burgers and fries when just across the street he could have just as easily gone to Starbucks instead and avoided the ravages of IR and obesity.

***

The Optimal Diet

What diet is best for health and longevity? As we saw earlier, many different societies have their own answer to this question. The Greek Monks at Mt. St. Athos have no recorded disease (other than 11 cases of prostate cancer.)[261] They swear by red wine, religious fasting, and a pesco-vegetarian diet. Similarly, those who practice the Mediterranean diet advocate lots of a vegetarian food with low meat except fish. They consume olive oil and enjoy moderate amounts of daily red wine. The Adventists mostly prefer a Lacto-ovo-vegetarian diet without coffee or wine.

My research and personal experience favors a variation of these: Lots of coffee and whey protein, TRE fasting, and resistive exercise combined with moderate red wine, and a Lacto-ovo-vegetarian approach. I believe this is best not only for health and longevity, but for lowering insulin levels, IR, and obesity. This approach also targets the two reasons why most fad diets fail: uncontrolled hunger and slowed metabolism.

THE OPTIMAL DIET: LACTO-MEDITERRANEAN

- Borrow the best from the St. Athos Monks: intermittent fasting; TRE 16 hour fasts x 4 days per week
- Borrow the best from the Adventists: Lacto-ovo-vegetarian diet
- Borrow the best from the Mediterranean Diet: liberal fish & olive oil & wine
- Borrow the best from the Coffee Cure: 4 cups of coffee per day
- Don't forget to add the whey and RT if you are actively trying to lose weight
- Adopt the best lifestyle: Daily fresh air, clean water, outdoor activity, and spirituality.

The Lacto-Mediterranean lifestyle dovetails with the Coffee Cure program. Stay outdoors each day, and be active. Hanging outside by the pool like Faith and I, or like the monks in their gardens, or simply fishing in the Mediterranean will all help you gain health. Belief in God or the practice of prayer or meditation is proven to lower your inflammation (CRP). Do it everyday. There is a reason Adventists and St. Athos Monks live longer, and its more than just diet and exercise.

With the Coffee Cure, no one can complain of uncontrolled appetite or cravings, and more importantly there is no yo-yo weight regain. Falling off the wagon is unheard of, unless one never finishes Phase I or refuses to drink coffee. Finally, no one can say the diet is difficult, unless they can't swallow coffee or they have pain with using stretch bands.

In that case, my answer would be that undergoing painful needle sticks each day to treat the alternative, diabetes, is more inconvenient and more painful than the Coffee Cure. Arthritic joint pain and rehabilitation following joint replacement surgery is even more painful. And swallowing the pain pills and anti-inflammatory medication is more complicated than drinking coffee and whey.

I have been on the Coffee Cure program for over six years now with the modification of my high volume RT. No yo-yo-ing. No temptation to stop it. It has become my habit and lifestyle. Today, my IR is under excellent control. My weight is never a problem. I like coffee and whey protein and I sip it all day long. My chest and arms are full and my waist is once again leaner. I have lots of energy and sleep like a rock. My cholesterol has dropped from 200 to 95. My triglycerides are down from 350 to 120. My blood sugar is down from 102 to 98. My HDL rose from 25 to 42. I can easily do a half dozen pull ups, the most of my life.

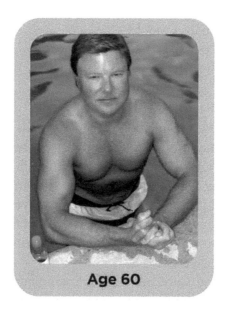

Age 60

I have tried all the fad diets and failed them. Low-fat failed because restricting fats while increasing starches and carbs worsens IR. It turns out that higher carbohydrates are even worse for people with IR. Carbohydrate entry is blocked into muscle and the sugar ends up at the liver where it is converted to fat, producing even more IR. Low carb diets failed me too. At first, I lost weight quickly with meat. Much like Byron, I craved greasy rotisserie chicken. I liked bacon. I craved the turkey skin on Thanksgiving. I figured it was healthy, but it turns out that low carb and high meat consumption can and does make one fat. The weight that I lost on low carb came off of my arms and legs. My waist stayed the same.

After a couple of years on low carb, I did not want anyone to see me in a tank top. I did all the wrong exercises. I lived on the Stairmaster. Everyday for years I did one hour a day. I saw no results. I looked the same. My blood pressure, sugar and inflammation stayed the same. Sure, I felt good after I did it, but I would go home and reward myself with more lousy food. Myoslacking will keep you fat. It was only when I learned how to get healthy that I started to change.

Now I eat clean six days a week with an emphasis on complex carbs like fruits and vegetables. Mediterranean or Adventist types of diets are associated with longevity. Low carb is fine with high protein, but not okay with high-fat. Try to keep saturated fat intake below 10%. Get your 10% saturated fat mainly from cheese and fermented dairy. Get your unsaturated fat mainly from fish, olive oil, and monounsaturated fats like nuts.

Don't believe anyone who tells you that saturated fats like grass-fed beef or coconut oil are healthy. Try to keep your total daily fats, unsaturated plus polyunsaturated below 30%. Drink coffee and whey protein to lower inflammation and curb your appetite. When eating fat, aim only for good fats such as those found in avocado, plants, fish, etc. Don't eat fats that are solid at room temperature. No tropical fats like palm oil. Reserve your unhealthy food for your cheat days. Don't overdo portion size when you cheat. Preload your cheat foods with coffee and whey.

The Coffee Cure diet is the result of my hard-fought experience at combining the best of the low carb, low-fat diet approach, while getting rid of the worst components. The best exercises, the resistive ones, I have found are low in resistance and high in volume. I would shoot for 20 sets of 20 repetitions everyday, which amounts to 400 muscle contractions.

RT exercises are easy to do anywhere. One does not need to change clothes, or sweat, or shower. One does not need to ride a bike, drive to a gym, or even get out of bed to do them. One can enjoy a benefit with as little as a 5 minute session, the proverbial "Five and Fly". It doesn't matter if you lift a gallon of water, a two-liter bottle or if you use ankle weights or if you prefer elastic bands. All of it is going to benefit you.

The studies on aerobics, unfortunately, show that it often promotes or causes inflammation. Calvacante's research shows that aerobic exercise promotes and can cause inflammation in up to 40% of the studies. RT does not. Resistance exercises are associated with most of the same benefits as aerobic exercise including lower blood pressure, lower post exercise blood pressures, and increases in basal metabolism.

Any exercise is better than none, though. One prospective study looked at two groups of women who were matched for bone density. One group was trained with RT for two years while the other group did not do RT. The back strength as measured in kilograms almost doubled in the RT group while it stayed nearly the same in the non-exercise group.[262]

Eight years later after both groups became sedentary; the exercise group still enjoyed an advantage of less than one-half of the fractures of the exercise group. The non-exercise group not only had weaker muscles, but had 2.7 times the number of fractures of the exercise group. Clearly, RT results in longer term improvements in metabolism, muscle mass, and resistance to sarcopenia that one does not enjoy with aerobic exercise.

The Coffee Cure Diet comprises the best of all the diets while eliminating the worst. It uses the best of exercises. It's perfect for the vast majority of my patients as well as our current Western society, especially those who suffer from insulin resistance and its related conditions.

***

How Much Health Do You Want?

I once asked my dentist, "Which teeth do I have to floss?"

He answered, "Only the ones you wish to keep."

So the real question for you is not "How much of the Coffee Cure program should I implement?" It is, "How much health do you want?" I see patients all the time who pick and choose and only do parts of the Coffee Cure. That's their choice. My role is to present the information, and it is your role to decide what you need.

***

"Anything new since your last appointment?" I asked my patient Joyce.

"Lost 18 pounds," she said.

"18 pounds?" I repeated.

"Yeah, I am drinking the coffee like you said I should."

"When do you drink it?" I asked, not remembering that she had started the program.

"Just before meals and when I wake up."

"Are you drinking whey protein too?"

"Yep, just like you said, 15 grams before each meal. It is hard to get it to dissolve in the coffee, but I manage to get it down. The stuff really works."

I was impressed with her weight loss, but more so by the noticeable decrease in the size of her right knee. Joyce had been a patient of mine for some 20 years and had struggled with obesity and bad knees. 18 pounds of weight loss on her 250-pound frame was not as apparent as her right knee going down from the size of a basketball to the size of a cantaloupe.

"So, how about the time-restricted eating?" I asked her.

"Say what?" she asked.

"You know, eating your meals in an eight-hour time frame."

"Now that is tough for me because I don't sleep well. I awaken all the time throughout the night. Sometimes I get a snack to help me fall asleep."

"Are you doing the exercises?" I asked.

"I walk to the mailbox and back and feed the horses and chickens," she replied. "My knees hurt too much to do any exercises."

Joyce is an example of someone who does only two of the four pillars, but none of the RT. She is forever stuck in Phase I. No diet changes. Yet, it always amazes me that even a little bit of the Coffee Cure goes a long way.

Many of my patients don't share my passion or urgency for reversing their metabolic syndrome. They are not so concerned about the stroke, heart attack, or cancer in the distant future. They are much more worried about their immediate concerns; joint pain, insomnia, and tending to the livestock.

Then you look at Byron deep into Phase III, committed to changing his diet and his daily exercises, committed to transforming himself. Byron, however, has faced death. He was wheeled into the operating room and told that he would be placed under anesthesia while his chest was cut open, and his heart was repaired. He was told that there was a chance that this would be his last conscious moment on earth, and there was a chance that he might not wake-up from the operation. Byron has told me many times, "I can't go back to eating normally unless I want to die. I have to make this work."

And me, why am I so OCD about staying a step ahead of the IR and the metabolic syndrome? Maybe it is because I have witnessed so many of my patients paying the price. Maybe it is because I have watched this movie so many times that I know the ending by heart.

Take my patient, Dale. He was a Merle Haggard look-alike. I treated his back pain for many years. He had a large grin and walked with a swagger. He had run a pool hall for most of his life and loved to display his gold chains and dazzling watch. He thought of himself as a ladies' man. He delighted in telling me tall tales about the time that he had won a man's $1000 in a pool match and then hustled him out of his Cadillac, yet had the heart to give him bus fare to get home.

Dale was a large man with a gut the size of a Thanksgiving turkey. I checked his labs; his blood pressure was elevated at 160/110. His cholesterol was 250 and his blood sugar was 115. His triglycerides were 300. I insisted on placing Dale on a diet. He refused. I referred him back to his family doctor for better blood sugar control. He started on necessary blood pressure and blood sugar medicines, but those could not compete with his terrible dietary habits and sedentary lifestyle.

"How much exercise do you do?" I asked.

"Well, I walk to the mailbox and back each day."

"What do you eat?" I asked.

"Oh, I eat fairly healthy you know, chicken and fish. I have cut down on my red meat."

"Dale, we have got to do something." I pleaded.

A couple of years later he had gained 30 more pounds. His belly was now the size of a watermelon and he was short of breath during his office visits.

"You have got to get your blood sugar down; it is up to 130, and you are developing diabetes. Your blood pressure is up to 170/120."

"Nope," he said. "I don't need to," he answered.

"Dale, you are not going to live much longer at this rate."

Dale and I were at the same age at age 58.

"Well, when it's your time, it's your time," he replied with a grin.

"See you next month," I said.

But next month Dale didn't show up. He finally came in six months later. Dale rolled in with a wheelchair with his right leg covered in a bandage. It had been amputated just above the knee joint.

"What happened?" I asked.

He replied, "Well, I had this sore that just didn't heal. Finally they had to amputate. Now I have to take these insulin injections and I have to be on a strict diet."

"When I asked you to go on a diet, you told me that you couldn't."

"Well, that was then, but after you lose your leg it changes your viewpoint," he said. "Now I have no choice."

Over the next year, Dale struggled with a non-healing above-the-knee amputation wound. It just wouldn't heal due to the diabetes, so we were unable to fit him with a prosthesis. Dale was unable to do any exercises as he was stuck in his wheelchair. He had lost copious muscle in his shoulder and chest while growing larger in the abdomen. He was aging decades before my eyes. He was developing new sores on his left foot, the only remaining good limb.

Within six months Dale stopped coming in altogether to his appointments. He had been hospitalized. His left leg had also been amputated, and he resided at a nursing home. I read about his death in the nursing home shortly before the age of 60.

Dale was robbed of at least 20 years due to his metabolic syndrome. He died way too young. At a minimum, Dale could have started drinking coffee and whey. He could have pulled on stretch bands and timed his meals. Even if he never changed his diet, he would have benefitted. This brings me to Kylie.

Just as I was completing this book, my patient Kylie died unexpectedly.

I first assumed Kylie's care when she was 29 years old. She stood 5 foot 3 inches tall and weighed in at 250 pounds. Her BMI was 44 and change. She was morbidly obese. But not in the normal proportion. She gained her weight chiefly in the abdomen, and suffered from classic metabolic syndrome. Both her parents suffered from obesity and diabetes, and the insulin-resistant genes were passed down to her.

She resisted diets. Her family was invested in ethnic dishes, and to them food meant love. Slowly, but consistently, year over year, she put on weight. She developed fatty liver, diabetes, thyroid cancer, all classic complications of insulin resistance. She developed knee arthritis and lower back pain from the inflammation.

By age 42 Kylie had put on 100 pounds, but was still able to walk with a cane and her grip was still up to 35 pounds. By age 46, she became bedridden at 480 pounds. Her muscle strength dropped as her body fat increased. Her grip had dropped to 15 pounds.

Insurance would not approve the recommended bariatric surgery due to her thyroid cancer. She developed kidney failure.

Kylie was hospitalized for some two months, and thankfully she lost about 170 pounds through a forced hospital diet. When she returned to see me, she appeared to be a transformed woman. "I won't gain the weight back. I promise," She vowed.

We talked about the importance of maintenance, and I gave her materials on the Coffee Cure Diet.

"I want you to start drinking coffee and whey immediately, "I stated.

"I don't know," she said.

When I called to confirm her appointment 2 weeks later, her mother answered. "Kylie died yesterday," She explained through tears. Subsequently, I learned she had died from a blood clot to her lungs, a pulmonary embolism. The risk is higher in those with insulin resistance.

Kylie was dead at age 49, just two months shy of her 50th birthday.

My heart sank. Kylie had died just at the very time she was beginning to turn her weight and insulin resistance around. But her time ran out. She should have lived to be a grandmother and made it into her eighties. The metabolic syndrome had robbed her of at least thirty years. It robbed Abby of ten years, and Dale of twenty.

My great regret is that I was too slow. I had twenty years with Kylie to figure it out. And I failed her.

The original title of this Chapter, the final one of the book, was "Live to 100". But now I recognize the goal is NOT to live longer. The real goal for my patients, and I, all those with insulin resistance, is to not get robbed, not to die before your time.

The Coffee Cure Diet is not burdensome; it involves drinking coffee and whey before meals as well as pulling on a few stretch bands and timing your meals.

I can't help but wonder if Abby had just started doing this five years ago, would she be coming down with pancreatic cancer today? With a daily dose of lactoferrin and lowering her insulin and blood sugar levels, I think not.

Would Kylie have continued to gain weight if at 350 pounds she had to swallow eight oz of coffee and 15 grams of whey before she sat down to dinner? I think not.

And finally what if Dale had beefed up his grip strength, fasted four days a week, and on top of that knocked down his blood triglycerides with whey protein at each meal? Would he still have been robbed? Maybe of a few years, but I will bet not twenty.

So, would I like to live to be 100? If I kept my mental faculties and didn't wind up in a care home, maybe.

But much more to the point, I don't want to get robbed of a normal life expectancy. I don't want to be surprised one day to hear that I have three or four months left.

So I say to you, all those who share the scourge of insulin resistance, "Don't worry so much about your diet. Make smart food choices most of the time, and enjoy your cheat day. But please at the very least, drink your coffee and whey each day. Keep up your muscle strength. And wait at least 16 hours before breakfast."

That is the real message of this book. "Failure to add your coffee and whey each time you add fuel may void your warranty of 80 years of life expectancy."

AFTERWORD

"Are these the shadows of the things that Will be, or are they the shadows of things that May be?"

– Charles Dickens, "A Christmas Carol"

When Dr. Gerald M. Reaven first proposed insulin resistance as the cause for Type II diabetes, he was disbelieved and even ridiculed by many skeptics. But Dr. Reaven persisted in his research, not accepting opinions, but instead, insisting upon facts, and only facts generated from well-controlled scientific studies. Then, in 1988, he dropped a bombshell with his famous Banting Lecture by linking high blood pressure, high blood sugar, and abnormal HDL and triglycerides together as Syndrome X, now known as Metabolic Syndrome. This condition is now an essential predictor of increased risk for heart disease, stroke, diabetes, and premature death.

Likewise, when Charles David Keeling measured carbon dioxide concentrations in the atmosphere, many thought his readings incorrect, and his predictions of global warming as "alarmist". Through years of meticulous research, however, Dr. Keeling was able to conclusively demonstrate that CO2 levels were higher than had been recorded since the dawn of human civilization, some 10,000 years earlier. Using carbon isotope fingerprinting, the extra CO2 was traced back to fossil fuel burning starting in the Industrial Revolution, but now rapidly accelerating. A graph of Dr. Keeling's results is now famously called the "Keeling Curve" and is displayed at the National Academy of Sciences in Washington D.C. By 2006, the Keeling Curve was approaching levels the earth had not seen in millions of years.

Now, in 2019, the evidence for climate change is no longer theoretical. It is in most people's faces. The El Niño floods, the La Niña droughts, the tsunamis, forest fires, hurricanes, cyclones, typhoons, melting sea ice, ocean dead zones, dying whales and polar bears, coastal floods, and extreme heat tell us this is not a dream; it is very real. Seventeen out of the hottest years in recorded weather have occurred in the past twenty years. The public now accepts that the climate is changing, and action may be required.

The reality is that we are destined to quickly go much higher, to levels that have not been seen on this planet for some twenty million years.

Projected Co2 Levels: Business as Usual Scenario:

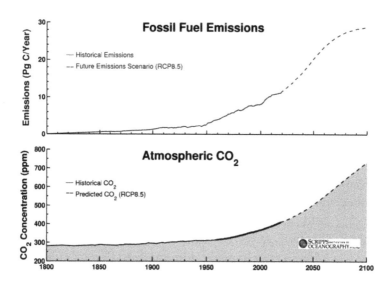

Figure 34. Courtesy of Scripps Institute of Oceanography

Fortunately, the world has sobered up, perhaps in the nick of time, and all major nations signed the Paris Agreement in 2015 promising to take voluntary action to curtail CO_2 emissions. Many countries are converting to solar or wind energy and electric cars. They are quickly phasing out fossil fuels. But the United Nations has also urged people to adopt a meatless diet. This can substantially reduce CO_2 emissions by more than 50% by the year 2050 according to the U.N. Agriculture, especially beef production, accounts for more carbon footprint than all the world's trains, planes and automobiles combined.

Projected C02 Level: Paris Changes & Meatless Diets Scenario:

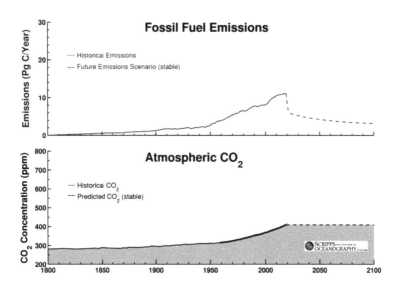

Figure 35. Courtesy of Scripps Institute of Oceanography

Several prominent groups have proposed variations of the Lacto-ovo-vegetarian diet that I favor. They advise little or no beef, and lots of nuts and fruit. The main criticism of such an approach is that people don't know how to transition smoothly and safely. The danger is they will substitute refined flour or processed food for the meat as I once did. Doing so can kill you if it sufficiently raises your TG/HDL ratio. The other danger is they will try it, find it too difficult, and give up, just like I also did. Using the Coffee Cure to transition to Lacto-Mediterraneanism is the best solution.

The Coffee Cure is the simplest, easiest, and healthiest way to slowly convert to a plant-based diet slowly, and can be done in stages. Some may stop the Coffee Cure in Phase II after adopting at least Meatless Mondays. Others may complete Phase III going three full days a week without meat. Many will reach Phase IV and enjoy meat only once a week on their cheat day.

My daughter has just reached this point. When she indulges in her formerly favorite turkey sausage, she becomes ill for three solid days. I suspect she and many other Phase IV Coffee Cure graduates, like myself, will simply swear off meat altogether, not because they must, but because their systems now reject it. In either of these scenarios, both you and the planet will benefit.

ACKNOWLEDGEMENTS

Many people have helped me complete this work. My transcriptionists, Della Bowman and Candice Barner, were constant allies. Della ended up shouldering the entire project when it came to the last five drafts. Thank you, Della. I could not have done this without you.

Dan Crissman, my editor, reviewed the manuscript cover-to-cover no less than three times. On the final review, he slashed and burned 30,000 words making this book readable. Allow me to thank my great artist at FIVERR, Danny Media, otherwise known as Daniel Ojedokun, a talented young man who designed the cover and color-coordinated all the charts within. Thanks to my cartoonist at FIVERR, who created the two fantasy maps. His FIVERR handle is Kitsunekei1 and also occasionally uses his real name Antonio Rafael Garcia Hernandez.

Thanks to my lawyers, David Sharifi and Justin Arel. I never realized how complicated Trademark and Corporate law were until they schooled me.

I appreciate all those researchers whose work I relied upon in this book. Thanks to Dr. Larry Beeson, Dr. Gary Fraser, Dr. P.K. Mills, and Dr. Michael Orlich for their work over the years with the Adventist Health Studies. Thanks to Dr. Ralph A. Defronzo for his pioneering work on insulin resistance and diabetes. Dr. Ancel Keyes deserves credit for his monumental research and development of the Mediterranean diet. Thanks to my friends at 48-Hour Book. I also appreciate all the feedback, support and cooperation of my many loyal patients. I appreciate the insight, inspiration, and unswerving support of my dedicated wife, Faith, without which this book would not have been written. Finally, and most importantly, I credit God as the guiding force in the completion of this project.

APPENDIX I:

FREQUENTLY ASKED QUESTIONS

1. **I cannot drink coffee because it upsets my stomach. Can I still lose weight with the Coffee Cure?** Absolutely, many of my patients have lost weight using only three of the four pillars of the Coffee Cure. If you eliminate coffee, but still employ whey protein, resistive training, and time-restricted eating you can be expected to lose weight.

2. **What exactly does the Coffee Cure "cure"?** It does not cure any specific disease; however, it helps you combat insulin resistance and the Western diet and lifestyle. Lowering your weight and insulin resistance will in turn lower your risk of contracting diabetes and its related diseases.

3. **Do I have to change my diet to do the Coffee Cure program?** Strictly speaking, you do not have to change your diet to employ the four pillars. That is the beauty of the Coffee Cure program. It is designed to allow people to lose weight in spite of the Western diet and lifestyle. With that being said, your weight loss and health progress will be much better if you strive to improve your nutrition.

4. **I have had a heart attack. Can I do the Coffee Cure program?** As I advise everyone get your doctors approval and permission before starting the Coffee Cure program or any diet for that matter. With that being said, the studies show heart disease risks are reduced with coffee. Patients who drink coffee have less risk of recurrent heart attack than those who do not. Those who perform intermittent fasting or time-restricted eating seem to have less inflammation and oxidative stress than those who do not. Survivors of heart attacks who perform low to moderate levels of resistive exercises tend to do better than those who do not. In general, the Coffee Cure is a very healthy approach regardless of your underlying condition, but specifically I would advise anyone to get medical clearance before beginning it.

5. **I have osteoporosis. Can I still do the Coffee Cure?** Again, I would obtain the consent and permission of your physician first, but the individual pillars of the Coffee Cure are conducive to bone health. The Korean study shows that coffee drinkers have denser bones than non-coffee drinkers. Those who do resistive exercises tend to have better bone density than those who do not. There are some studies that suggest whey protein, by improving muscle mass has a secondary effect on bone density.

6. **I have had bariatric surgery. Can I still do the Coffee Cure?** Once again, I would recommend you obtain permission from your doctor. With that being said, whey protein is a routinely recommended supplement for post-bariatric surgery patients. The studies are clear that whey protein helps bariatric patients in their quest for protein and adequate nutrition. Exercise is always a good recommendation especially if done in moderation and with your doctor's supervision. Bariatric patients are particularly vulnerable to the development of fractures in the long bones and the development of osteoporosis. Therefore, resistive exercise makes a lot of sense.

7. **Can I still use Himalayan salt while I am on the Coffee Cure?** The ideal daily salt intake remains controversial. However, from the standpoint of simple weight loss, it is a good rule of thumb to keep your salt intake moderated and under 5 grams a day. Studies, however, seem to show that with extremely low salt intake, there is an increased rate of disease probably from stimulation of the renin angiotensin aldosterone system. I am not advocating anyone avoid salt altogether. I believe the lowest point of the J-shaped risk curve is between 2 and 5 grams of salt per day. It does not matter, in my view, if it is Himalayan salt, Sea salt, or Rock salt. Salt should have iodine added to it.

8. **Can I still use coconut oil on the Coffee Cure?** Coconut oil has a high saturated fat content despite the marketing efforts to pass it off as a medium change triglyceride, which it is not. The simple answer is that coconut oil is a solid at room temperature and for that reason it is a favorite of food manufacturers as it gives it resistance to rancidification and a long shelf life. However, I would view coconut oil as I view saturated fat; not as bad for you as simple sugar and not as bad for you as trans fats, but still not healthy.

9. **I cannot do the time-restricted eating. I get low blood sugar after about 12 hours. Can I still benefit from the Coffee Cure program?** Once again, if one does three out of the four pillars, one can do well on the Coffee Cure program. Certainly, if you comply closely with the coffee and whey pillars as well as the resistance training pillar, you could do well even without the time-restricted eating pillar. With that being said, I have not encountered anyone who was unable to work up to the 16-hour fasts. If you eat properly during the eight-hour period, consume enough polyunsaturated fats, protein, and fibrous vegetables, you should be able to hold out without attacks of low blood sugar. If you supplement during the fasting period with whey protein shakes, this will provide the calories that should prevent any hypoglycemic attacks.

10. **I do not want to get bands or dumb bells. I walk my dog regularly, isn't that enough?** Treadmill walking or walking ones dog are good low-intensity exercises, but they will not in my experience reverse insulin resistance to the extent that resistive training will. Resistive training has a host of other benefits as well, including improving bone density, muscle mass, preventing sarcopenia, etc. It also stimulates the production of anti-inflammatory myokines. All of this is not done to any significant degree by walking the dog or walking the treadmill.

11. **I work 80-hours a week and do not have the time or energy to fast or do any exercise. Can I still do the program?** When one gets down to giving up two pillars, and only performing two pillars, the results are less predictable. Certainly, I have seen patients who have benefited from performing only one pillar of the program such as supplementing with whey protein before each meal. However, two pillars are much better, and four pillars are what I consider necessary to achieve weight loss and health success. Although, I appreciate the sacrifice of working 80-hours a week and not having the motivation to stick to an exercise or diet regimen, the Coffee Cure is so easy that I cannot image one not being able to do at least four pillars. Simply try fasting periods of 12-hours the first couple of weeks and then increase these to 13-hours the next couple of weeks, and then gradually with the use of whey protein during the fasts increase them to 14-hours. I have not encountered patients who were unable to improve their fasting duration with this approach.

12. **I read that aerobic exercise burns more fat than resistive training. Why should I do resistive training when aerobics will help me lose weight quicker?** Aerobic training can burn more calories per session. However, it is not as convenient and it certainly does not produce the benefits to muscle and bone that resistive training does. It is much more important to be consistent and to perform exercises five and six days a week than to do a longer aerobic session only once or twice a week. I know. I tried it, and for many years daily treadmill exercises of even an hour five to six days a week simply did not provide me the progress that the shorter sessions of resistive training did.

13. **I prefer soy protein over whey. Can I simply do that instead?** There are many types of protein as I have discussed in the book. There are different varieties of vegetable protein such as pea protein, rice protein, and soy. There are different varieties of animal protein such as beef, chicken, and milk protein. However, whey protein has unique benefits. It is a natural ACE inhibitor. This confers upon it ACE inhibitor or anti-hypertensive activity which is particularly beneficial for those with IR, and this sets it apart from all other proteins. It contains lactoferrin. This gives it anti-bacterial, anti-viral, and anti-tumor activity. It also enhances the immune system. It also tends to suppress appetite and increase secretion of incretins such as GLP-1 and CCK both of which have been shown to regrow cells in the pancreas and in the brain. And it is a powerful anti-oxidant.

14. **I prefer green tea over coffee. Can I substitute green tea?** The short answer is that green tea, although being a powerful anti-oxidant, does not have all of the benefits of coffee. However, it is quite healthy and I would not be upset if someone substituted green tea for coffee and did the other four pillars of the program. Certainly using only three pillars is enough to benefit and substituting green tea for coffee is essentially like using three and on-half pillars of the program.

15. **I read that fasting lowers insulin levels better than the Coffee Cure. Is that true?** Popular books have come out advocating the benefits of fasting. Most of these books draw on the parallels with animal studies that show fasting tends to reduce the risk of cancer and promote longevity. Fasting is equated by some scientists as a form of caloric restriction which has definitely been correlated with longevity.

However, fasting in someone with IR, which is the majority of overweight patients in our country and in many cases around the world is associated with IR. That is, a normal person who fasts might experience increased IR after 72-hours while an IR person who fasts would experience increased IR after only 12-hours. The fasting can make the underlying IR worse which can worsen the underlying inflammation, oxidation, and weight gain process. Therefore, I recommend the abbreviated version of fasting known as time-restricted eating. I believe that this, in combination with resistive therapy, gives the best of both worlds to an overweight person with IR.

16. **I enjoy grass-fed beef. Is it as safe as fish or chicken?** Studies show that grass fed beef tends to have a lower saturated fat content than traditional grain fed beef. However, with that being said, beef is still beef, and it still contains saturated fat. Saturated fat can form free fatty acids after ingestion by an insulin-resistant person and free fatty acids can propel or exacerbate insulin resistance. Fish is a bit safer provided one obtains less than 37% of ones daily calories from fat. I refer to fish and chicken as a "garbage diet" in the book. Some may feel this is unfair. However, it is based on my own bitter personal experience. It is also based on my experience with patients, many who have gone on to develop heart attacks, strokes, dementia, and amputations, and early death with a diet of "fish and chicken." I strongly recommend IR individuals follow all four pillars of the Coffee Cure program as described in the book with their doctor's permission.

17. **I crave salt. How bad exactly is salt for you? I read that it is controversial and some health experts recommend salt.** Salt certainly is one of the fad recommendations these days along with prolonged fasts and coconut oil. However, the studies are fairly clear that high doses of salt are universally unhealthy for a person. They increase inflammation and aggravate hypertension. Most overweight people have IR and should avoid consuming too much salt. Very low intakes of salt can activate the renin angiotensin aldosterone system, but this is not a usual occurrence. Therefore, I do not recommend salt intakes of under 2 grams per day. Not enough salt is almost never a problem. Too much salt is a problem much of the time.

18. I crave sugar and cannot seem to hold out to my cheat day. What can I do? The best answer is to be patient and continue the Coffee Cure program. Most of my patients find that as their insulin resistance improves and their weight drops, they get better and better at holding out for the cheat day. Their cravings lessen because leptin resistance lessens along with the insulin resistance.

19. My blood pressure is only elevated when I go to my doctor. At home it is always normal. Should I worry? As I described in the book, I also have white coat hypertension. It developed when I was 18-years-old. At first I lived in denial believing that my blood pressure couldn't hurt me as long as it was normal when I took it at home. However, people must live in the world, and if the doctor's office can trigger hypertension, so can work or social situations. White coat syndrome is considered one of the first signs of insulin resistance and it has been demonstrated to pose a risk for end-organ damage. So, white count syndrome should be taken seriously.

20. My cholesterol and blood sugar are perfect. Do I still need to worry about insulin resistance? Insulin resistance is a very subtle process and can begin with only one of the factors such as a thick waist or high triglycerides. Even if one's cholesterol and blood sugar are normal, one can still have grossly elevated levels of insulin due to insulin resistance. These grossly elevated levels of insulin place one at great risk for heart disease and cancer in spite of normal blood sugar and cholesterol. Therefore, I think it is a good practice to use all four pillars of the Coffee Cure if there is any doubt or sign of insulin resistance such as a thick waist, high triglycerides, low HDL, white coat hypertension, etc.

21. I am of normal weight, blood sugar, and blood pressure. My cholesterol is perfect (low) except for high triglycerides of 250 and a low HDL of 38. Should I worry? Once again I would refer you to the prior question. If there is any sign whatsoever of beginnings of insulin resistance, I would employ all four pillars of the Coffee Cure. Your goal will be to normalize your weight, your insulin resistance, your waist, and maximize your nutrition. This would mean going on a plant-based diet similar to the Mediterranean or the Adventist diet, staying active, and essentially following the recommendations of the entire book.

22. **I am of normal weight, blood pressure, triglycerides, HDL, except that I gain all my weight in the middle. Do I still need the Coffee Cure diet?** Again, any sign of insulin resistance could mean that you have high levels of insulin. To be healthy you would want to abandon most of the Western diet and lifestyle using the Coffee Cure as a tool. Your goal will be to be on a plant-based diet with high levels of polyphenol intake, low levels of inflammation and oxidation.

23. **I do not want muscles and I do not want to look manly. I want to be feminine. I am afraid that I will end up looking like a body builder with the Coffee Cure with all this bulking up on whey protein and weight lifting.** Bulking up on whey protein is a myth. Most patients who employ the Coffee Cure actually get smaller and lighter. Muscle is denser than fat so the same weight of muscle will be smaller than the same weight of fat. Those who exercise muscle will not necessarily enlarge their muscle, but will look younger, smaller, and can actually look less masculine.

24. **Can I just drink my coffee in the morning and do two scoops of whey protein when I awaken?** The Coffee Cure program four pillars are all about timing. If one does not follow the timing, then one can lose most of the benefit. Drinking coffee in the morning and not before meals does not help the post-meal killer microns or sugar shards. In other words, it does not help reduce inflammation and oxidation, or triglyceride levels, or blood sugar levels. Similarly, in not taking whey protein before meals, one loses the appetite suppressant benefits. In order for the Coffee Cure program to be effective, each and every meal must be preceded by coffee and whey protein.

25. **I like my whey protein mixed in with blueberries in my morning fruit smoothie. Is that okay?** Mixing concentrated sugar, even fruit sugar, in with whey protein tends to counteract the benefit of the whey protein. The idea is to use whey protein to lower your post-meal blood sugar and blood fat surges. By adding blueberries to the whey protein shake, you are increasing the blood sugar surge. It is sort of like throwing gasoline and water on the fire at the same time. It is better than throwing just gasoline, but it will not have the same beneficial effect on insulin resistance and weight loss.

26. **I need my meat. Can I still do the rest of the Coffee Cure and benefit?** It depends. Certain types of meat are much, much worse than other types of meat. For example, fried bacon or fast food burgers are the worst as they contain trans fats and high levels of sodium. When one consumes both high levels of trans fats and high levels of sodium in one meal, one is asking for trouble. That is a tall order for even the Coffee Cure to help fight. However, if one is talking about a backyard BBQ with chicken taking care not to char the meat, then we are not talking about trans fats, and we are not talking about added sodium. If you must have meats, make sure that they are not prepared in restaurants or from fast food establishments. There is just too great a risk of trans fats and added salt. Although I hate the term "sticking with chicken and fish" as long as they are prepared trans-fat free in the supervision of your own home, they are probably okay. Do not ever believe that fish fillets prepared in a fast food outlet are safe as they are loaded with both trans fats and salts. I have learned to stay away from them even on my cheat day.

27. **I have cancer. Will the Coffee Cure help me?** The Coffee Cure is not a cure for cancer. Period. However, I strongly believe that those who perform all four pillars of the Coffee Cure and lose weight are reducing their risks of developing cancer, as well as other inflammatory and oxidative related diseases. That being said, if you have cancer or are a cancer survivor, I would run the program past your doctor and get his approval first. Certainly, there are good studies on many of the pillars of the Coffee Cure, that they can be beneficial in cancer survivors. The studies that stand out are the time-restricted eating studies where cancer recurrence was at least 50-70% less in those who fasted more than 13 hours compared to those who fasted less than 13 hours. Some studies suggest that whey protein can increase levels of glutathione which is an anti-oxidant. There have been some studies utilizing whey protein in patients with cancer. I am referring to the studies using lactoferrin as a form of non-toxic chemotherapy. Caloric restriction and fasting have been employed in the treatment of cancer with good benefit. Simulated fasting has also been employed in the treatment of cancer with good benefit. There is some evidence that fasting 24-48 hours before chemotherapy heightens the effectiveness of the chemotherapy. In summary, the Coffee Cure does not cure cancer. However, the individual pillars of the Coffee Cure have been shown in many scientific studies to have a

preventative effect against many inflammatory and oxidative diseases including some cancers.

APPENDIX II

MYTHS & MISCONCEPTIONS

1. **Coffee is unhealthy.** Caffeine by itself taken as an extract may be unhealthy, but the caffeine taken in the form of coffee is abundantly healthy as the 1000 or so natural compounds contained in coffee more than make up for any negative effect of the caffeine. Many studies show that coffee is not health subtractive, but overall is health additive. Coffee drinking is associated with lowering all-cause mortality. In general, coffee may help one live longer, but there is no evidence that it will shorten your life.

2. **Coffee is an addictive habit.** Addiction is usually defined as a compulsion that causes one harm in some way. In that vein, coffee drinking may become a habit. It usually does no harm, although I am sure that someone could come up with an argument in rare circumstances that it could contribute to stomach upset, rebound headaches, jitters, etc. By far, our unhealthiest national habits are addictions to sugars, sweets, fats, and salt; i.e. fast foods and processed foods. These are proven to be unhealthy. It is these habits that critics should concern themselves with, not coffee drinking. Additional unhealthy Western habits include sitting, marathon internet sessions, preoccupation with social media, cell phone addiction, texting while driving, etc. Some children today barely see the light of day much less get any exercise. Our best hope of breaking these habits that define the Western diet and lifestyle which is now a worldwide problem is to utilize a strategy that is both practical and effective. Adopting the four pillars of the Coffee Cure will steer people into a life of healthy fasting, plant-based foods, and increased activity. I believe the Coffee Cure is the tool that people will use to break their Western diet and lifestyle disease-producing habits.

3. **Coffee raises blood pressure.** No; caffeine raises blood pressure. Coffee lowers blood pressure over time.

4. **Coffee causes heart palpitations.** No; caffeine causes heart palpitations. Coffee actually lowers the chance of atrial and ventricular arrhythmias over time and reduces the risk of sudden cardiac death.

5. **Coffee dehydrates.** No; only people who are not used to coffee experience drinking associated dehydration. After a few days of tolerance, coffee hydrates a person almost as well as pure water.

6. **Coffee raises cholesterol.** No; only unfiltered coffee raises cholesterol, filtered coffee does not.

7. **Using the Coffee Cure means that one must drink coffee.** No, use of the Coffee Cure constitutes adopting at least three of the four pillars of the Coffee Cure program. My experiences show that following three of the four pillars produces excellent results. Coffee drinking represents only one pillar. It is possible for a person to lose weight and get healthy using only the non-coffee pillars of the Coffee Cure such as resistive therapy, time-restricted eating, and whey protein supplementation.

8. **The Coffee Cure sounds like a high protein fad diet due to the requirement of supplemental whey protein.** No, I recommend four or five 15 gram servings of whey protein per day. This represents 60-75 grams of whey protein which translates into 300 calories, less than 10-15% of total calories. Most nutritionists recommend up to 35% of total calories coming from protein. I do not recommend the discontinuation of any macronutrients. My advice is simply one of gradually adopting a plant-based diet such as the Adventist or Mediterranean over the typical Western diet. These recommendations do not constitute a fad diet.

9. **I hear too much coffee in some studies is associated with stroke and osteoporosis.** I do not advise more than four 8 ounce cups of coffee per day. This is considered moderate coffee drinking. Studies on moderate coffee drinking and bone density are mixed, although the Korean studies show coffee to improve bone density. When the pillars of whey protein supplementation and strength training are added, the Coffee Cure program decidedly improves bone health. Shifting to a plant-based diet, lowering insulin resistance, and

keeping coffee to less than or equal to four cups per day should not increase one's overall risk for stroke.

10. **Although most studies show a reduced risk of cancer with coffee, some old studies suggested increased risks for lung and bladder cancer with coffee.** The studies that showed increased risks were those not corrected for smoking. When risks for smoking are controlled, there is not an increased risk of any cancer. The modern studies look at "never smokers" who drink coffee to get the true data.

11. **Much has been made of the effect of hot liquid on throat cancer. Does coffee increase this risk?** I prefer my coffee cold or lukewarm anyway. The cooler you drink it, the safer. The hot liquid cancer risk applies to any liquid that you drink hot, not just coffee. I advise cooling it off before you consume it.

12. **You claim that aerobic exercise can increase inflammation and contribute to heart failure. That cannot be true.** I do not personally claim that. The studies tend to show that exercise involving oxygen in high-intensity produces oxidation which is only logical. However, low to moderate intensity exercise shows much less of that effect. I personally feel that low to moderate intensity aerobic exercise is fine and healthy. I would, however, avoid performing more than 3500-4000 calories of aerobic exercise per week. Dr. Ralph Paffenbarger researched and discussed the life-shortening effects and increased levels of oxidation associated with such excessive exercise.

13. **Aerobic training is superior to strength training.** They are both healthier than being sedentary. I find resistive training much easier to adopt for most people. Resistive training lends itself to exercise snacking such as five-minute intervals or taking stretch bands to the office or use while commuting. You simply cannot perform these aerobic activities as easily on the go or in small increments. It is easier to build a habit if you can start small. It is much harder getting a person to start bicycling, jogging, or going to the gym than using stretch bands. Today we have some 150 million Americans who have become insulin-resistant and at extreme risk for osteoporosis and sarcopenia. Aerobic exercise will not stop these conditions, but resistive training, if properly applied, will.

14. **Advising people to take up alcohol use is irresponsible.** I advise only red wine and in moderate amounts which equals one glass a day for women and two glasses a day for men with your doctor's approval and only in those who are insulin-resistant. I do not recommend hard liquor or beer and I do not recommend individuals take up drinking if they are not insulin-resistant. Alcohol drinking is not a formal part of the Coffee Cure, that is, it is not one of the pillars. It is associated with a thinner waist, lower weight, lower blood sugar, and a lower levels of insulin resistance, inflammation, and oxidation. Many healthy diets including the Mediterranean have reflected the proven benefits of polyphenol-rich red wine. It is effective against the components of the metabolic syndrome which has now become a worldwide crisis.

APPENDIX III:

THE SHOPPING LIST

Once you've mastered Phases I and II, Phases III and IV will help you master the Lacto-Mediterranean lifestyle, the goal of the Coffee Cure. With the improvements you will have noticed in the mirror and your health, you will want to take the next step. The next step is renouncing processed and fast foods as well as harmful foods such as meats.

The recommendations in this shopping list are a first step to change your grocery purchases. This is an important move toward the Lacto-Mediterranean lifestyle: a transformation from unhealthy habits to those of health. A return to 19th century eating routines when fast foods, high fructose corn syrup, preservatives and plentiful meats were not available. I recommend it for those of you who wish to adopt a healthier lifestyle, more of an Adventist/Mediterranean lifestyle that can add years to your lives. This shopping list helps prevent unhealthy or junk food purchases. If it is not on the list, you simply do not purchase it.

 "If it's not in the house, I can't eat it" is the principle I live by, and it works. If you wish to eat like an Adventist, and gain the Adventist health advantage, and the additional seven or eight years of life most Adventists enjoy, then use our shopping list whenever you buy food or groceries.

I. Produce

- Vegetables (all except potatoes). Emphasize cauliflower, broccoli, brussels sprouts or cruciferous vegetables. Include tomatoes, cucumbers, radishes, squash, sprouts, etc.
- Prepackaged salads including kale (we prefer the Eat Smart Sweet Kale) variety of Asian salads
- Sundried tomatoes
- Fresh beans
- Kidney Beans
- Mushrooms (use as meat substitute)
- Cabbage, all types
- Lettuce, all types (We prefer as a bread replacement for use in open-face sandwiches.)

- Peppers (Stuff with turkey meat once a week.)
- Avocados (Make a breakfast with toast.)
- Fruits (We prefer apples and tangerines daily.)
- Nectarines
- Cantaloupe (Serve with cottage cheese for breakfast.)
- Grapes
- Tofu

II. Poultry and Dairy

- Ground turkey (For once a week or less – makes great stuffed peppers and haystacks.)
- Shredded cheese (Prefer low-fat such as mozzarella or Swiss but a mixture including a small amount of cheddar is okay.)
- Coffee creamer (Prefer low or no sugar. Best is our own KC.)
- Sliced cheese (Prefer Swiss, dry or a low-fat version.)
- Cottage cheese
- Sour cream
- Eggs
- Butter (Use natural sparingly. Avoid sprays or margarines.)
- Parmesan cheese
- Nutritional yeast powder (and/or flaxseed meal) for serving over toast and butter
- Whipped cream (for use with frozen blueberries)

III. Fish

- Salmon
- Tuna (water packed, not packed in oil)

IV. Snacks and Soda

- All variety of nuts except macadamia and cashews (Prefer peanuts, pistachios, walnuts, almonds.)
- Chips (For cheat days. Avoid regular use.)
- Bottled water

V. <u>Cans and Jars</u>

- Vegetarian chili beans (Make sure no lard or meat is contained in the ingredients.)
- S&W chili beans (Pinto beans with chili peppers, onions, garlic, and zesty tomato sauce.)
- Vegetarian refried beans (We prefer Market Essentials and fat free.)
- Garbanzo beans
- Jalapeno stewed tomatoes
- Canned corn
- Kimchi

VI. <u>Condiments</u>

- Balsamic vinegar
- Bar-B-Que sauce (Avoid high fructose corn syrup.)
- Olive oil
- Olives
- Salsa
- Peanut butter (Natural in oil. Prefer Adams.)
- Hot peppers & Pepperoncinis
- Ketchup (Organic; has no high fructose corn syrup.)
- Mustard

VII. <u>Beverages</u>

- Coffee, all types, decaffeinated and caffeinated
- Tea (Prefer chamomile and green)

VIII. <u>Frozen foods</u>

- Frozen vegetables
- Frozen fruits (Prefer blueberries.)

IX. <u>Breads, Crackers and Chips</u>

- All fermented types: Sourdough and rye bread.
- Bagels (Only occasionally.)
- Crackers (Only occasionally, prefer Triscuits. We combine with Kimchi, hot mustard and Swiss cheese.)

- Tortilla Chips (Only occasionally, prefer Trader Joe's brands. Lower sodium better.)

X. Foods to avoid*

- Seafood is acceptable as long as there are fins and scales. Recommend against shrimp, lobster, or clams. These are bottom feeders or scavengers that concentrate toxins. Almost all the world's fish are contaminated with mercury. Therefore advise fish maximum at one serving per week. Prefer wild-caught Alaskan types.
- Meat. Generally we avoid meat of all types, whether it is chicken, fish, or beef. If you must have meat, then limit to one or two servings a week, preferably only fish or organic turkey.
- Would recommend against beef and against pork. Beef and pork are highly insulinogenic.
- Avoid fowl that are raised with hormones and arsenic such as conventional chickens.
- Avoid birds that have been scavengers.
- We prefer to eat occasional duck, pheasant, or turkey.
- Processed meat.
- Recommend against all lunch meat even those that say "no preservatives" due to high concentrations of sodium and other chemicals.
- Avoid salami, jerky, or any colored preserved meats as they are usually loaded with nitrates which are highly carcinogenic.
- No deli lunch meats.
- No smoked meats.
- No colored meats.
- No ham.
- No pork.
- Crackers, cookies, and cereal. Recommend against all of these in general due to the presence of hydrogenated oils as a preservative. These play havoc with cholesterol and are unhealthy.
- I recommend against any products containing high fructose corn syrup. If one must have treats on a cheat day, then do so sparingly. Would prefer any types of cookies or candies or cereals that were in existence prior to 1960 as they have the least sophisticated preservatives and sugars.

- Homemade desserts are probably safer (if made without Crisco or shortening). Would still limit them to cheat days one or two days each weekend.
- Would recommend against cakes, frostings, and ice cream as they contain health-defeating combinations of fat and sugar. Reserve for your cheat day.
- Dark chocolate is better than milk chocolate.
- If you must eat sugar, try to eat it without fat and if one must eat fat, try to eat it without sugar.
- Also, limit all unhealthy foods to small and limited proportions and only consume on cheat days.
- Avoid coconut or palm oil. Notice the food industry is now using these in place of trans fats and hydrogenated oils for shelf stability. Read the labels when purchasing cookies, pastries, health bars, etc.

*Remember the worse the food, the more important it is to pre-load with whey and coffee.

GLOSSARY

Abductor Leg Exercises: Abductor leg muscles are a group of muscles on the outside of the hip used to bring the knees apart.

Above the Knee Amputation: The surgical removal of a limb above the knee joint.

ACE inhibitor: Angiotensin-converting enzyme inhibitor. These are prescription drugs like lisinopril and captopril, but can also refer to natural substances like whey protein.

Adductor Leg Exercises: Adductor muscles of the hip are a group of muscles used to bring the thighs together.

Adenosine Receptor: A class of G-protein receptors with adenosine as a ligand. There are four known types of adenosine receptors in humans; A1, A2A, A2B, and A3. Each are encoded by a different gene. The adenosine receptors are commonly known for their antagonist's caffeine and theophylline whose actions produce the stimulating effects of coffee, tea, and chocolate. Adenosine receptors have various functions throughout the central nervous system, heart, and lungs.

Adenovirus Infection: The most common cause of illness in the respiratory system, but they can also cause eye, bladder, and GI infections.

Adipokines: Hormones secreted by visceral fat cells also known as signaling proteins secreted by adipose tissue typically pro-inflammatory cytokines such as TNF-alpha and IL-6 where anti-inflammatory cytokines such as adiponectin or other cytokines such as leptin.

Adiponectin: A signaling protein secreted by adipose tissue involved in regulating glucose level.

Adventism: A branch of protestant Christianity started in the United States approximately 1843 to 1844.

Adventist Health Study: A series of long term medical research projects of Loma Linda University with the intent to measure the link between lifestyle, diet, disease, and mortality of Seventh-Day Adventists. The first study is known as the Adventists Mortality Study extending from 1960-1965 reflecting that Adventist men live 6.2 years longer than non-Adventist men and that Adventist women had a 3.7 year advantage of their counter parts based on life table analyses. The Adventist Health Study-1 was conducted between 1974 and 1988 finding that Adventist men lived 7.3 years longer and Adventist women lived 4.4 years longer than other Californians. The Adventist Health Study-2 began in 2002 and was run by Dr. Gary Fraser and a team of researchers at Loma Linda University School of Medicine and funded by the National Cancer Institute. Among other things, it revealed a vegetarian diet pattern that was associated with a more favorable health profile and a lower risk of metabolic syndrome.

Aerobic Exercise: Physical exercise of low to high-intensity that depends primarily on aerobic energy. It is also known as endurance training. It includes running, jogging, swimming, and cycling.

Age Spots: Benign spotty discolorations in the skin ranging from brown to black, occurring mostly in older than age 50 adults, resulting from ultraviolet skin damage.

Aldosterone: A steroid hormone produced in the adrenal gland. It helps conserve and retain sodium through the kidneys, salivary glands, sweat glands, and colon. It plays a central role in the regulation of blood pressure as well as sodium and potassium levels.

Alzheimer's Disease: Dementing disease characterized by neurofibrillary tangles and deposits of beta-amyloid. Apolipoproteins enhance breakdown of amyloid in most people, but those with inherited APOE4 iso-forms are at high risk for the disease because of failure of the apolipoproteins to break down the amyloid.

AMP Kinase: 5-adenosine monophosphate activated protein kinase is an enzyme that promotes use of fat and glucose when cellular energy is low.

Amyloid Plaque: These are aggregates of proteins that become folded into a shape that allows many copies of the proteins to stick together forming fibrils. In the human body, amyloids have been linked to the development of various neurodegenerative diseases including Alzheimer's disease.

Ancel Keys: A Minnesota physiologist who studied the effects of both under-nutrition and over-nutrition. He is famous for work on starvation and the adverse effects of dietary saturated fat. The first scientist to champion the Mediterranean Diet.

ANGI-II: Abbreviation for angiotensin II.

Angiotensin: A peptid hormone that causes vasoconstriction and an increase in blood pressure. It is part of the renin angiotensin system which regulates blood pressure. Angiotensin also stimulates the release of aldosterone from the adrenal cortex to promote sodium retention by the kidneys.

Anti-inflammatory: An anti-inflammatory is the property of a substance or treatment that reduces inflammation or swelling.

Antioxidant: Compounds that inhibit or decrease oxidation. Oxidation is a chemical reaction that can produce free radicles thereby leading to chain reactions that may damage the cells of organisms. Antioxidant defenses help balance the oxidative state of plants and animals through a complex system of overlapping enzymes such as catalase and superoxide dismutase produced internally.

Aorta: Large vessel that carries blood away from the left ventricle.

Apoptosis: A form of programmed cell death that occurs in multicellular organisms which includes cell shrinkage, chromatin condensation, and decay. The average adult human loses between 50 and 70 billion cells each day due to apoptosis. Organisms that lack efficient apoptosis ability have a higher risk for many diseases. Insufficient apoptosis can result in uncontrolled cell proliferation such as cancer.

Apple Cider Vinegar: Vinegar made from fermented apple juice and used in salad dressings, marinades, vinaigrettes, food preservatives, and chutneys. It is made by crushing apples and then squeezing out the juice. Bacteria and yeast are added to the liquid to start the alcoholic fermentation process which converts the sugars to alcohol.

ARB: This is also known as an angiotensin-II receptor blocker and modulates the activity of the renin angiotensin system. They are similar to ACE inhibitors as they are pharmacological agents used as first-line antihypertensives in patients who have developed hypertension. ARBs appear to produce less adverse effects compared to ACE inhibitors.

ARC: Refers to the arculate nucleus of the hypothalamus which is an aggregation of neurons. These govern factors possible for hypothalamic function involved in appetite.

Arrhythmia: This is a group of conditions in which the heartbeat is irregular, too fast, or too slow.

AS-160: A widely expressed activating protein which plays a role in mediating insulin action. Insulin stimulation of Glut-4 is dependent on AS-160.

Ascites: The accumulation of fluid within the peritoneal cavity causing abdominal swelling.

Asthma: Common long term inflammatory disease of the airways of the lungs. It is characterized by variable symptoms including reversible airway obstruction and symptoms of wheezing, coughing, chest tightness, and shortness of breath.

Atheroma: Also known as an atheromatous plaque which is an abnormal accumulation of material in the inner layer of the wall of an artery; it is present in the arteries of most adults. The material consists mostly of macrophage cells or debris containing lipids, calcium, and a variable amount of fibrous connective tissue. The accumulated material forms a swelling in the artery wall which may intrude into the channel of the artery, narrowing it, and restricting blood flow. Atheroma is the pathologic basis for the disease entity atherosclerosis, a sub-type of arteriosclerosis.

Atherosclerosis: Disease in which arteries progressively narrow due to pathologic build up of plaque usually associated with inflammation.

Atkins Diet: A weight-loss program devised by Robert Atkins. It is classified as a low carbohydrate diet.

Atrial Fibrillation: Abnormal heart beat rhythm characterized by rapid and irregular beating of the atria.

Autoimmune Disease: Condition arising from an abnormal immune response often against a particular body part.

Autophagy: The natural regulated mechanism of the cell which disposes of unnecessary dysfunctional components.

Balloon Angioplasty: Use of an inflatable balloon catheter to treat narrowed arteries (usually of the heart).

Bariatric Surgery: Operation that involves removing or shortening some of the stomach or small intestines to reduce nutrient absorption and promote weight loss.

Basal Cell Carcinoma (BCC): Also known as basal cell cancer. It is the most common type of skin cancer and appears as a painless raised area of skin which may present with ulceration or small vessels running over it. It grows slowly and can damage the tissue around it, but it is unlikely to spread to distant areas or to result in death.

Ben Taub Hospital: Teaching hospital of Baylor College of Medicine and one of the busiest trauma centers in the United States.

Beta-amyloid: Involves peptides of 36-43 amino acids that are crucially involved in Alzheimer's disease as the main component of the amyloid plaques found in the brains of Alzheimer's patients. These are derived from amyloid precursor protein (APP) which ultimately form oligomers.

Beta Cells: A type of cell found in pancreatic islets that secrete insulin and amylin. Beta cells make up 50-70% of the cells in human islets. In patients with type I or type II diabetes, beta cell mass and function are diminished leading to insufficient insulin secretion and hyperglycemia.

Biomarker: A measure or indicator of some biological state or condition. One common biomarker is PSA (prostatic specific antigen). Markers are useful in the medical diagnostics for colon, breast, lung cancer, and melanoma.

Blood Brain Barrier: A highly selective semipermeable border that separates the circulating blood from the brain and extra cellular fluid in the central nervous system. The system allows the passage of some molecules by passive diffusion as well as selective transport of glucose, water, and amino acids that are crucial to neural function. It restricts the passage of pathogens or large or hydrophilic molecules into the cerebral spinal fluid while allowing the diffusion of hydrophobic molecules such as O_2, CO_2, and hormones.   Cells of the barrier actively transport metabolic products such as glucose across the barrier using specific transport proteins.

Blood Culture: Microbiological culture of the blood.

Body Mass Index (BMI): A value derived from mass and height of an individual. The BMI is defined as the body mass divided by the square of the body height and is universally expressed in units of kg/m^2.

Borderline Blood Sugar or Pre-Diabetes: Stage before diabetes mellitus in which not all of the symptoms require to diagnose diabetes are present, but blood sugar is abnormally high.

Brain Derived Neurotropic Factor (BDNF): A protein that is encoded by the BDNF gene. This helps to support survival of existing neurons and encourage the growth and development of new neurons. It is active in the various areas of the brain including the hippocampus cortex and basal forebrain which are areas vital to learning, memory, and higher thinking.

Bronchodilator: Substance that dilates the bronchi and bronchioles decreasing resistance in the airway and increasing air flow to the lungs.   Common bronchodilators include Salbutamol (albuterol) and Terbutaline.

Byetta: A medication used to treat diabetes mellitus type II. It is often used together with diet, exercise, and potential other anti-diabetic medications. It works by binding to intact glucagon-like peptid I (GLP-1) receptors.   The mechanism of action is to release more appropriate amounts of insulin following eating to suppress the pancreatic release of glucagon, to slow down gastric emptying, and produce a prolonged effect on reducing appetite known as satiety. Byetta reduces liver fat content and can help reduce accumulation in non-alcoholic fatty liver disease.

Bypass Surgery: A procedure designed to reroute flow through a blocked blood vessel.

Caffeic acid: Organic compound classified as a hydroxy-cinnamic acid. It is found in all plants because it is a key intermediate in the biosynthesis of lignan, one of the principle components of woody plant biomass and residues. Cinnamic acid is also found at a modest level in coffee.

Caffeine: Central nervous system stimulant of the methylxanthine class. It has several mechanisms of action, the most prominent of which is to reversibly block the action of adenosine on its receptor which consequently prevents the onset of drowsiness induced by adenosine. Caffeine also stimulates portions of the autonomic nervous system. It is known as a methylxanthine alkaloid. It is found in the seeds, nuts, or leaves of a number of plants native to Africa, East Asia, and South America as it helps protect them against predatory insects. The most well-known source of caffeine is the coffee bean. Beverages containing caffeine are ingested to relieve or prevent drowsiness and improve performance.

Cancer: A group of diseases involving abnormal cell growth with the potential to invade or spread to other parts of the body. These contrast with benign tumors which do not spread. Possible signs and symptoms include: a lump, abnormal bleeding, prolonged cough, unexplained weight loss, and a change in bowel movements. There are over a hundred types of cancers affecting humans. Most cancers can be prevented by not smoking, maintaining a health weight, not drinking too much alcohol, eating plenty of vegetables, fruits, and whole grains, vaccination against certain infectious diseases, not eating too much processed and red meat, and avoiding too much sunlight exposure.

Carbohydrate: Macronutrient consisting of carbon, hydrogen, and oxygen atoms. It contains 4 calories/gram and supplies energy. Complex carbohydrates are slow digesting compared to simple carbohydrates such as sugar found in candy, jams, and desserts which are rapidly absorbed.

Cardiomyocyte: A cardiac muscle cell. Each cell contains myofibrils. Like skeletal muscle cells, the majority of cardiomyocytes contain only one nucleus. They have a high mitochondrial density which allows them to produce ATP quickly, making them highly resistant to fatigue.

Casein: A protein found in milk. It comprises between 25-45% of the proteins in human milk.

Cataract: Clouding of the lens in the eye which leads to a decrease in vision. They can develop slowly and occur generally in older age. Symptoms include faded color, blurry vision, halos around lights, and trouble seeing at night. They are usually caused by aging, but can also be due to trauma, radiation exposure, or from accelerated oxidation.

Celebrex: A brand name for celecoxib. It is a Cox-II selective nonsteroid anti-inflammatory (NSAID). It is used to treat pain and inflammation of osteoarthritis and acute pain in adults.

Cell Adhesion Molecule (CAM): A subset of adhesion proteins located on the cells surface. Cell adhesion molecules help cells stick to each other and to their surroundings and are involved in the formation of atheromas.

Cheat Day: Slang term used to describe the one day each week that dietary restrictions are lifted to allow a broader selection of food intake; often used to denote one or two cheat meals within the day.

Chlorogenic Acid: A compound contained in coffee. It has been investigated for anti-inflammatory effects. It is present in the flesh of egg plants, peaches, and prunes.

Chlorogenic Acid Stimulated Glucose Transport: Chlorogenic acid in coffee stimulates skeletal muscle uptake of glucose by raising AMPK, adenosine monophosphate kinase through phosphorylation via both insulin and non-insulin dependent mechanisms.

Cholecystokinin (CCK): An incretin peptide secreted by the intestinal L-cells.

Cholesterol: A sterol molecule, a type of lipid. It is a building block of steroid hormones, bile acids, and vitamin D. According to the lipid hypothesis, there are multiple forms of cholesterol contained in the human body including LDL, IDL, VLDL, and HDL.

Chylomicron: Lipoprotein particles consisting of triglycerides (85-92%), phospholipids (6-12%), cholesterol (1-3%), and proteins (1-2%). They transport dietary lipids from the intestines to other locations in the body.

Cinnamic Acid: Component of caffeic acid and quinnic acid functioning as an intermediate in lignan biosynthesis.

Circadian rhythm: Any biologic process that displays an endogenous oscillation of about 24 hours. These are driven by a circadian clock and have been widely observed in plants and animals.

Cirrhosis: Condition in which the liver does not function properly due to long term damage. This damage is characterized by replacement of normal liver tissue by scar tissue. Causes include alcohol and long term fatty liver disease.

CKK: See cholecystokinin.

Clean Eating: Eating whole foods in their most natural state and avoiding processed foods such as refined sugars or those chemically preserved.

Clostridium Difficile: The organism responsible for C. difficile colitis (usually due to overuse of antibiotics).

Coarctation of the Aorta: A congenital conditioning where the aorta is narrow. This can result in rebound hypertension; one of the few correctable causes of hypertension.

Coconut Oil: Edible oil extracted from the kernel or meat of mature coconuts harvested from the coconut palm. Because of its high saturated fat content it is slow to oxidize and thus resistant to rancidification, lasting up to six months at $75\,^{\circ}$F without spoiling. Coconut oil is comprised of a combination of caprylic saturated C8 fatty acids, decanoic saturated C10 fatty acid, as well as lauric saturated C12 fatty acid, myristic saturated C14 fatty acid, palmitic saturated C16 fatty acid, and oleic monounsaturated C18:1 fatty acid. Coconut oil is thus approximately 99% fat and composed mainly of saturated fat (82% of the total).

Coffee Cure Diet with the Four Pillars: Weight-loss program with 1) coffee before each meal, 2) whey protein before each meal, 3) time restricted feeding, and 4) resistive exercises daily.

Coffee Cure Keto Style: See Lactoketo diet.

COPD (Chronic Obstructive Pulmonary Disease): A combination of chronic bronchitis and emphysema. It is known as a type of obstructive lung disease characterized by long term breathing problems and poor air flow. Symptoms include shortness of breath and cough with productive sputum. It is a progressive disease.

Copeptin: 39 amino acid long peptide and a preprohormone of vasopressin. Arginine vasopressin (AVP) also known as antidiuretic hormone (ADH) and is involved in multiple cardiovascular and renal pathways. Abnormal levels of AVP are associated with various diseases.

Coronary Arteries: The arteries of the coronary circulation which transport blood into and out of the cardiac muscle. These arteries include the left coronary, left anterior descending, the right coronary, and the circumflex coronary artery.

Coronary Artery Bypass Surgery (CABG): Also known as heart bypass. It is a surgical procedure to restore normal blood flow to an obstructed or narrowed coronary artery. Veins or other vessels are sewn to the coronary to circumvent or bypass the area of obstruction.

CRP: C-reactive protein. A protein marker that rises with inflammation. A protein found in plasma whose circulating concentrations rise in response to inflammation. CRP is synthesized in the liver in response to factors released by macrophages and fat cells (adipocytes).

Cystic Fibrosis: Genetic disorder that affects lungs, pancreas, liver, kidneys, and intestine. Long term issues include difficulty breathing and coughing up mucus as a result of frequent lung infections.

Cysteine: An amino acid with a thiol sidechain which participates in enzymatic reaction. Cysteine is instrumental in the synthesis of glutathione.

Cytokines: Signaling hormone proteins secreted by various body structures including atherosclerotic plaques, beta-amyloid plaques, and visceral fat.

Cytokine Theory: The hypothesis that depression and related symptoms are reflective of proinflammatory cytokines and deregulation of immune mediators.

DASH (Dietary Approaches to Stop Hypertension): Program promoted by the National Heart, Lung, and Blood Vessel Institute, part of the NIH and an agency of the United States Department of Health. DASH is rich in fruits, vegetables, whole grains, and low-fat dairy.

Dead Lift: Straight leg exercise where weight is lifted off of the ground to the level of the hips and then lowered again.

Deadly Quartet: Group of symptoms also known as metabolic syndrome or syndrome X.

Defibrillator: Device for cardiac resuscitation that delivers electrical current (counter shock).

Dementia: Group of symptoms associated with decline in memory or thinking skills severe enough to interfere with everyday activities. Alzheimer's disease accounts for 60-80% of these cases.

Diabetes: A disease characterized by inadequate or ineffective insulin action which impairs the ability to regulate blood glucose.

Dopamine: Neurotransmitter and catecholamine. Used in the treatment of heart failure and shock.

Diabetic Gangrene: Skin infection in the limb of a diabetic that often spreads into the bloodstream and can result in amputation, sepsis, or death.

Echovirus: Type of RNA virus that belongs to the Enterovirus B group. It is typically found in the gastrointestinal tract.

End Organ Damage: Refers to damage to major organs fed by the circulatory system such as heart, kidneys, brain, and eyes due to uncontrolled hypertension.

Endotoxin: Part of the outer wall of gram negative bacteria; also known as LPS.

Endurance Training (ET): A form of aerobic training such as sustained running, cycling, and swimming, also known as aerobic training. Distinguished from resistive training which is usually anaerobic.

Energy Drink: Carbonated or non-carbonated sweetened beverage with added stimulants and supplements; usually sugar and caffeine promoted to improve concentration and stamina. It is often falsely promoted as being healthy.

Epinephrine: Also known as adrenaline. It is a medication and a hormone. As a medication it is used to treat a number of conditions including anaphylaxis, cardiac arrest, and superficial bleeding. It is produced normally by the adrenal glands and certain neurons and plays a role in the fight-or-flight response.

Escherichia Coli: A gram negative rod-shaped anaerobic bacteria found in the lower intestinal tracts of warm blooded animals.

Fad Diet: Weight-loss approach promoting quick weight loss, usually with highly restrictive food choices and often associated with negative health consequences.

Fats: A macronutrients containing nine calories/gram broken down during digestion and metabolism into free fatty acids. Can be used for fat storage or burned for energy.

Fatty Infiltration of the Liver: Also known as hepatic steatosis. Fatty liver disease is where excess fat builds up in the liver and can produce inflammation leading to scarring or cirrhosis.

Fermented dairy: Cultured milk products such as cheese, yogurt, cottage cheese, and sour cream.

FEV-1:   The forced expiratory volume in one second. It is the volume of air that can be forcibly blown out in one second after full inspiration.

Fibrin cap: The top of an atheroma composed of macrophages, foam cells, and dead cells. It is prone to rupture and can produce thrombosis or vessel blockage.

Fibrosis: Scar tissue.

Fibrous Cap: Layer of cells including muscles, macrophage, foam cells, lymphocytes that represent the final step in the formation of an atheroma.

Fibrous Carbs: Energy sparse nutrient containing relatively more fiber than calories. Examples include; broccoli, brussels sprouts, kale.

FMD (Flow-mediated Dilation): Widening of the arteries in response to increased blood flow.

Foam Cell: Fat laden macrophage that marks the early stages of atherosclerosis.

Forensic Pathologist: Medical specialist that performs autopsies.

Free Fatty Acid: The digested products of fat when not contained as part of a triglyceride. When circulating in free form in the blood they are toxic and can produce skeletal muscle resistance within four hours. They are increased in most obese individuals.

FVC: Forced vital capacity. It is the volume of air that can be forcibly blown out after a full inspiration.

G6Pase   Glucose-6-phosphatase is the enzyme that breaks G6P, glucose-6-phosphate, into one free glucose and one phosphate molecule. It marks the final step in gluconeogenesis.

Garbage Diet: Slang term for the phrase "less red meat and more fish and chicken" as it usually denotes a diet filled with junk food, saturated and trans fats.

Gastric Emptying: The process of food transiting from the stomach to the small intestine.

GERD: Gastroesophageal reflux disease; a long term condition in which stomach contents rise up into the esophagus resulting in either symptoms or complications. Symptoms include the taste of the acid in the back of the mouth, heartburn, bad breath, chest pain, vomiting, breathing problems, and wearing away of the teeth. Complications include esophagitis, esophageal stricture, and Barrett's esophagus. Strategies to avoid include not lying down within three hours after eating, raising the head of the bed, losing weight, avoiding foods which result in symptoms, and stopping smoking.

GLP-1:   Glucagon like peptid I. An incretin peptide secreted by intestinal L-cells.

GLP-1 Raising Drugs: These belong to a class known as incretin mimetics used to treat diabetes. Examples include; Byetta and Victoza.

Glucagon: Protein hormone secreted by pancreas after eating to promote an increase in blood sugar.

Glycemic Index: A number on a scale of 1-100 reflecting the rate of blood sugar elevation caused by carbohydrate consumption. Low is 55 or less, and high is 70 or more. The higher the index the more rapid the insulin response.

Glycogen: Storage form of glucose found within muscles and liver. Unlike fat, deposits of glycogen are non-toxic and do not secrete cytokines.

Gluconeogenesis: The process of producing glucose from fats or amino acids. It allows the brain to obtain glucose during times of fasting. The pathway is somewhat blocked by the drug Metformin.

Glutathione: Antioxidant capable of preventing damage by free radicals.

GMP (Glycomacropeptide): A component of whey protein.

Gram Negative Organism: A particularly harmful type of bacteria with characteristic cell envelopes comprised of lipopolysaccharides (LPS) that can cause septic shock.

Gram Negative Septic Shock: The potentially fatal medical condition that occurs when sepsis leads to dangerously low blood pressure and abnormalities in cellular metabolism. The modern mortality rate of septic shock runs approximately 25-50%.

Goiter: A swelling in the neck usually resulting in a swollen thyroid gland due to dysfunction from iodine deficiency.

Gut Incretin: A group of metabolic proteins that stimulate a decrease in blood glucose levels.

Heart attack: an event where there is sudden cessation of blood flow to an area of the heart usually due to an embolism or thrombosis with result in tissue death; also known as myocardial infarction or simply MI.

Heart Enlargement: Otherwise known as cardiomegaly or pathological enlargement of the heart typically in response to long standing high blood pressure.

Helicobacter pylori: Previously known as campylobacter pylori, this is a gram negative organism found in the stomach. It is linked to the development of duodenal ulcers and cancer.

Hemoglobin A1C: The percentage of hemoglobin bound to glucose. It corresponds to ones average blood sugar level over the last 30-90 days.

Hepatic Jaundice: The yellowish pigment of the skin and sclera of the eyes due to high bilirubin levels usually related to liver, pancreatic disease, or cancer.

Herpes Simplex: Viral infection caused by the herpes simplex virus characterized by small blisters often seen as cold sores.

HDL: High density lipoprotein. Unlike the larger LDL or VLDL that deliver fat molecules to cells, the HDL particles do the reverse. They remove fat molecules from cells and this can result in reducing fat within artery wall atheromas causing regression of atherosclerosis.

Heavy Metal: Dense metal noted for its potent toxicity. Examples include cadmium, lead, and mercury.

High Blood Pressure: Also known as hypertension. This is a long term medical condition in which the blood pressure in the arteries is persistently elevated. Typically it produces no symptoms, but in the long term can cause numerous diseases such as stroke, heart failure, coronary disease, cardiac enlargement, kidney disease, dementia, peripheral vascular disease, and vision loss.

High Fructose Corn Syrup: Sweetener made from corn starch which leads to an unfavorable lipid profile and blood sugar regulation.

Human Parainfluenza Virus: Viruses of approximately 150-250 ng in size. The second most common cause of hospitalization in children under age 5 suffering from respiratory illness.

Hydrogenated Oil: An oil that can be chemically hydrogenated by adding hydrogen to an unsaturated double-bond converting it to a single-bond. Similar to trans fat.

Hypothalamus: Part of the brain that helps regulate hunger, temperature, thirst, fatigue, and circadian rhythms.

Idiopathic Hypertension: The form of hypertension or high blood pressure that has no identifiable cause.

IL-1: A proinflammatory cytokine also known as interleukin-1.

IL-6: A cytokine that can act both as a proinflammatory cytokine or an anti-inflammatory myokine, also known as interleukin-6.

Inflammation: Complex response to injury involving heat, pain, redness, and loss of function. Chronic inflammation can cause damage and loss of tissue.

Inflammatory Cytokine: Signaling molecule that promotes inflammation.

Insulin: Hormone secreted by pancreas in response to carbohydrate consumption. It is necessary for muscles to absorb glucose.

Insulin-Like Growth Factor-1 (IGF-1): A structurally-similar protein to insulin with similar anabolic properties.

Insulin Resistance (IR): The pathological condition in which cells fail to respond normally to the hormone insulin. This results in a compensatory over-secretion of insulin which can lead to an atherosclerotic cholesterol profile, high blood pressure, diabetes, obesity, and related diseases.

Insulin Sensitive Muscle: The condition where insulin triggers skeletal muscle glucose uptake easily.

Insulin Sensitivity: The rate at which the body can process insulin.

Intestinal Permeability: Refers to the filtering ability of the absorptive surfaces of the intestines. The intestine normally exhibits some permeability allowing nutrients to pass through the gut while maintaining a barrier to keep potentially harmful substances such as LPS from leaving the intestine and migrating to the body more widely. Mucosal barrier participates in intestinal permeability.

IMCL (Intramyocellular Lipid): A marker for insulin resistance refers to microscopic abnormal deposits of fat within muscle.

IVP (Intravenous Pyelogram): The radiographic procedure used to visualize abnormalities of the urinary system.

J Shaped Risk Reduction: A risk curve where risk initially falls with low value of the variable and then rises with the high value. Examples include: Health risk of alcohol consumption and health risk of salt consumption.

KC: abbreviation for Koffee Cure.

Killer Microns: Sang term for elevated chylomicrons. These are post-meal blood fats that can damage health.

Lacto Ovo Vegetarian: Type of vegetarian that also consumes dairy and eggs.

Lactoferrin: A component of whey protein that has multiple beneficial effects. It is used for treating stomach and intestinal ulcers, diarrhea, and hepatitis C. It is used as an antioxidant and it is protective against bacterial and viral infections. It also stimulates the immune system preventing tissue damage related to aging, promoting healthy intestinal bacteria, and helping to prevent cancer and regulating the body processes iron. Other names include apo-lactoferrin, bovine lactoferrin, human lactoferrin. Lactoferrin helps to regulate the absorption of iron in the intestine. It helps to protect against bacterial infection possibly by preventing the growth of bacteria by depriving them of the central nutrients or killing bacteria by destroying their cell walls. It is active against infections caused by some viruses and fungi. Involved in the regulation of bone marrow function (myelopoiesis) and the ability to boost the bodies immune defenses.

Lacto Keto Diet: Low carbohydrate diet usually under 75 grams per day combined with lacto ovo vegetarian.

Lacto Mediterranean Diet: The Mediterranean diet with the addition of moderate cheese and eggs.

Lactose: The main sugar found in milk or dairy products.

Latissimus Dorsi Muscle: Large flat muscle that stretches the sides behind both arms.

LDL: Low density lipoprotein. LDL delivers fat molecules to cells and can drive atherosclerosis if they become oxidized and embedded in the walls of arteries.

Leaky Gut Syndrome: Slang term for increased intestinal permeability.

Leg Lift: Exercise which strengthens abdomen and hip flexor muscles.

Legumes: Beans such as kidney, navy, pinto, lentils, garbanzo, or chick peas: The fruit or seed of the fabaceae (leguminosae) family.

Leptin: A hormone produced by adipose cells that acts on the hypothalamus receptors to suppress hunger.

Leptin Resistance: The condition of sustained high Leptin levels which produces an insensitivity to hunger suppression by the brain.

Lisinopril: A blood pressure reducing medication that works by blocking the angiotensin or ACE system, the system involving angiotensin-converting enzyme.

Liver Glucose Production: Generation of glucose by liver from non-carbohydrate sources, also known as gluconeogenesis.

Low Carbohydrate Diet: One that causes weight loss by restricting carbohydrates. Examples include keto, paleo, and coffee cure keto style.

Low-Fat Diet: Used to describe a diet containing less than the normal amount of dietary fat i.e. < 20-25%.

Low HDL: Low levels of HDL or high density lipoproteins are a form of dyslipidemia and recognized risk factor for numerous diseases related to atherosclerosis.

LPS: Lipopolysaccharide also known as lipoglycan and endotoxin found in the outer membrane of gram negative bacteria.

Macrophage: A type of white blood cell that engulfs and digests cellular debris. Examples include Macrophage type I and Macrophage type II.

Marine Resiliency Study: The Marine resiliency study is a collaborate project with an objective to provide an early analysis of predictors of mental health outcome such as posttraumatic stress in the Marines.

Mediterranean Diet: Diet high in legumes, olive oil, fruits, and vegetables; moderate in fish and low in dairy. It is moderate in wine and low in non-fish meat.

Melanoma: Tumor of the melanocytes (pigment containing cells). A form of skin cancer.

Metabolic Syndrome: A condition with three of the following: large waist, high blood pressure, high blood sugar, high cholesterol, or high triglycerides usually associated with obesity or overweight.

Meta Analysis: Statistical analysis that combines the results of multiple scientific studies. Meta analyses can be performed when there are multiple scientific studies addressing the same question with each study reporting measurements that are expected to have some degree of error.

Metastasis: Refers to the spread of cancer cells from the original tissue to other parts of the body.

Moderate to Low Red Wine Intake: This refers to one glass of wine per day (115 ml or 5oz) for women and two glasses of wine a day for men (300 ml or 10 oz) which are considered safe by most healthcare practitioners.

Modified Pushup: Pushup with knees as the pivot point.

Monounsaturated Fats: A triglyceride in which most of the fatty acids have one point of un-saturation.

Mortality Study: A scientific analysis of the effect on the death rate by a selective variable. Examples would be: Coffee drinking or metformin use, which both decrease all cause mortality.

Mount St. Athos Greek Monks: Members of the Eastern Orthodox Church and one of the 20 monasteries in the Mt. St. Athos location distinguished by their healthy lifestyle and low rate of disease.

mTOR: Mammalian target of rapamycin which is a regulator of metabolism.

Muscle Sink: Slang term used to simplify the complex biochemical process of insulin's action on skeletal muscle and glucose absorption.

Myoslacker: Slang term used to describe one who avoids resistive exercises, and suffers from either sarcopenia or low muscle mass. This often co-exists with persistent insulin resistance.

N6 Polyunsaturated Fatty Acid (N6PUFA): Fatty acid with an unsaturated bond at the N6 position. It can be pro-inflammatory or anti-inflammatory.

Nautilus Equipment: A variety of fitness equipment.

Neurodegeneration: This is the progressive loss of structure or function of the neurons including the death of neurons. Many neurodegenerative diseases include amyotrophic lateral sclerosis (Lou Gehrig's disease), Parkinson's disease, Alzheimer's disease, and Huntington's chorea.

Neurodegenerative Diseases: Alzheimer's and Parkinsonism, and progressive diseases of the brain and central nervous system thought to be accelerated by oxidative (free radical) stress.

Neuroinflammation: Inflammation of the central nervous system which usually includes microglia or brain and spinal cord. It can be initiated due to a wide variety of causes including infection, traumatic brain injury, or autoimmunity. Inflammation of the central nervous system is abnormal and associated with neurodegenerative diseases highly related to insulin resistance.

Omega III: Polyunsaturated fatty acid also known as Omega III PUFA.

Open Heart Surgery: Coronary artery bypass graft surgery.

Osteoarthritis: Degenerative condition involving breakdown of joint cartilage and then underlying bone.

Osteoblast: Bone producing cluster of cells.

Osteoclast: A cell that breaks down bone tissue.

Oxidation: Chemical reaction in which electrons are lost.

Oxidative Damage: Toxic effects to cells through production of peroxides or free radicles often causing damage to DNA.

Oxidative Disease: Disease is accelerated by free radical damage i.e. Alzheimer's, Parkinsonism, atherosclerosis, cancer.

Oxidized LDL: A harmful type of LDL cholesterol produced when normal LDL is damaged by free radicals.

Palm Oil: Tropical oil, one of the few saturated vegetable fats. It is semi-solid at room temperature. It is prized in the food industry because of its lower cost and longer shelf-life. It is resistant to rancidification. It is made from the pulp of the fruit of the oil palm. Tropical oils are proinflammatory and pro-oxidative.

Parkinson's Disease: Long term neurodegenerative condition with shaking, rigidity, and slowness of movement and difficulty with walking.

Pathological Heart Involvement: Disease of heart related to pathology of muscle or electrical system.

Pericardial fat: Form of visceral fat surrounding heart.

Pesco-Vegetarian: The practice of a diet that includes fish or sea food, but not the flesh of animals.

Pheochromocytoma (PCC): A neuroendocrine tumor of the medulla of the adrenal glands that secretes high amounts of catecholamines mostly norepinephrine. This results in elevated heart rate, flank pain, palpitations, and blood pressure. It is one of the few causes of hypertension that can be corrected. A pheochromocytoma crisis is rare but potentially life threatening.

Phytochemical: Chemical produced by plants to help them compete, survive, or thrive.

Pilates: Form of movement muscle therapy.

Polyphenol: Anti-oxidant containing polyphenol structure and often found in nature.

Post-meal Chylomicron: Triglyceride rich cholesterol protein that transports dietary fats through the bloodstream.

Postprandial: After meal.

PPAR Gamma: Peroxisome proliferator activated receptor gamma; regulates fat storage and glucose metabolism.

Prebiotics: Compounds in food that induce growth of beneficial microorganisms.

Pre-Diabetes: The condition if impaired insulin action or insulin resistance that results in inadequate glucose regulation and elevated fasting blood sugar usually within the 100-125 range.

Prilosec: A proton-pump inhibitor antacid.

Probiotics: Live microorganisms intended to provide health benefits when consumed.

Processed Food Vegetarian: Slang use of vegetarianism alluding to the process of avoiding meats by consuming energy-dense processed food such as simple sugars and saturated and trans fat; an unhealthy diet.

Protein: Macronutrient containing four calories/gram. They are broken down during digestion and metabolism into amino acids. They are used for building muscles and protein. They are not stored but can be converted to sugar through gluconeogenesis.

Pseudomonas: Gram negative bacteria considered an opportunistic human pathogen.

PTSD: Post traumatic stress disorder. Emotional disorder triggered by traumatic event.

Pubmed: A free search engine accessing the medline data bases of references or abstracts on the life sciences or biomedical topics.

Pull-ups: Upper body compound pulling exercise.

Pulmonary Artery: The artery that transports deoxygenated blood from the right side of the heart to the lungs, vessel that carries blood into the lungs for oxygenation.

Pulmonary Embolism (PE): Blockage of an artery in the lungs by a substance that has moved from elsewhere in the body through the bloodstream, usually a blood clot from the leg (deep venous thrombosis). Symptoms may include shortness of breath, chest pain, and coughing up blood. Severe cases can lead to passing out, abnormally low blood pressure, and sudden death.

RAAS: The Rennin-angiotensin-aldosterone-system.

Refined Carbohydrate: A food consisting mainly of carbohydrate without the natural fiber that slows the release of sugar. These tend to promote rapid rises in blood sugar and consequently rapid rises and over-production of insulin. Usually a processed food.

Renin: Hormone precursor to angiotensin I and II. A potent vasoconstrictor and stimulator of catecholamine release.

Reperfusion: Restoration of blood flow to an organ or tissue after being blocked.

Resistive Exercise: Also known as strength training (ST or RT). It is a type of exercise that specializes in the use of resistance to induce muscular contraction to build strength and size of skeletal muscles. It is considered an anaerobic activity.

Resistive Training (RT): The form of exercise involving repetitive contraction of muscles. This builds volume and strength in muscle. It also stimulates myokine secretion.

Respiratory Syncytial Virus: Also known as human orthopneumovirus that causes respiratory tract infections. Very common infant infection.

Rotavirus: The most common cause of diarrheal disease among infants and young children.

Salt: A mineral containing sodium and chloride.

Salt-Sensitive Hypertension: High salt intake that raises blood pressure in salt-sensitive individuals.

Salmonella: A rod-shaped gram negative bacteria of the enterobacteria family. It can be involved in typhoid fever.

Sarcopenia: The degenerative loss of skeletal muscle usually at 1% per year beginning after age 50.

Satiety Hormone: A hormone such as GLP-1 or CKK which slows gastric emptying and provides satiety signals to the hypothalamus of the brain. An incretin.

Saturated Fats: Unhealthy fats that are solid at room temperature. They are pro-inflammatory and promote diseases of oxidation and aging such as heart disease, cancer, and dementia.

Seated Curl Biceps Exercise: Contraction done while sitting.

Second Hand Smoke: Environmental tobacco smoke contamination.

Seventh-Day Adventist: A Protestant Church denomination distinguished by its observance of Saturday as the Sabbath as well as practicing a vegetarian diet.

Shift Work: An eight-hour work schedule that overlaps the typical sleep cycle.

Shigella: Gram negative aerobic rod-shaped bacteria closely related to E.coli. Leading causes of bacteria and related deaths worldwide.

Skeletal Muscle Insulin Resistance: The suppression or failure of the limb muscles to rapidly absorb glucose.

Soluble Fiber: Healthy plant food that cannot be completely broken down by human digestion. It delays gastric emptying which improves glucose absorption.

Squamous Cell Skin Cancer: One of the three main types of skin cancer; the other two being melanoma and basal cell. Spread or metastasis is more likely than in basal cell.

Starchy Carbs: Energy-dense nutrient containing up to three times as much carbohydrate than fibrous carbohydrates. Usually found in potatoes, legumes, and rice.

Stent: A metal or plastic tube inserted into a blood vessel to keep it open.

Stroke: The sudden cessation of blood flow to an area of the brain by thrombus, embolism, or bursting of a blood vessel (hemorrhage).

Sudden Cardiac Death: Sudden cessation of effective blood flow due to heart disease resulting in cardiac arrest.

Sugar Jelly: Slang term for glycogen.

Sugar Shards: Slang term for elevated post-meal blood sugars that can damage health.

Supine: Laying horizontal with face and body pointed upward.

Swiss Exercise Ball: Air filled ball of elastic PVC between 14 and 34 inches in diameter used in physical therapy and training.

Syndrome X: A group of symptoms also known as the deadly quartet. Modernly it is referred to as the Metabolic syndrome

Tai Chi: An internal Chinese martial art practiced for both its defensive training, its health benefits, and meditation.

Take Shape for Life: Subsidiary for Medifast involving meal replacements for weight loss.

Textured Vegetable Protein: A deflated soy flour product, a byproduct of extracting soy bean oil. A highly processed vegetable food.

TG/HDL Ratio: Otherwise known as the triglyceride to HDL ratio. It is a ratio strongly correlated with cardiovascular disease. It is a risk factor for myocardial infarction and stroke.

Thermic Effect: The amount of energy required to digest and metabolize a macronutrient. A greater thermic effect raises basal metabolism, the amount of calories the one burns while resting.

Third Hand Smoke: Contamination by tobacco smoke that lingers following extinguishing of the cigarettes, cigar, or tobacco product.

Thymine Dimers: Molecular lesion formed from thymine or cytosine bases in DNA caused by ultraviolet damage. These dimers are the primary cause of melanoma in humans.

Time Restricted Eating (TRE): Also known as time restricted feeding. Refers to a particular type of intermittent fasting where an individual compresses their meals into a narrower window. Restricted feeding of 16-hours refers to eating all ones meals within an 8 hour window allowing 16 hour daily fast.

Time Restricted Feeding (TRF): Consuming ones daily food intake within a window of less than 24 hours. A typical TRF paradigm involves consuming food in an eight-hour window allowing a 16-hour fast.

TLR-2:   Toll-like receptor 2 that plays a signaling role in the immune system and inflammation.

TLR-4:   Toll-like receptor 4, a signaling protein involved in triggering inflammatory cytokines and immune response.

TNF-alpha: A cell signaling protein (cytokine) involved in inflammation.

Toxic Visceral Fat: Fat in the peritoneal cavity in the abdomen located between organs that secrete inflammatory cytokines.

Trans Fats: Vegetable fats that are hydrogenated by processing to produce more desirable physical characteristics i.e. solid at room temperature, longer shelf life. However, they are associated with adverse health effects such as high levels of inflammation, heart disease, and cardiovascular disease.

Triceps Bench Dip Exercise: A medium intensity exercise that uses body weight to contract the triceps; also known as a chair dip.

Triceps Kick-Back Exercise: Triceps extension exercise performed while leaning forward usually resting on one knee.

Trigonelline: An alkaloid produced by many plants found in coffee.

Triglycerides: A molecule consisting of glycerol and three fatty acids designed as a way to transport fats within the bloodstream.

Tropical Oil: Coconut and palm oil.

TRX System: Otherwise known as the Total Resistive Exercise system; a form of strength training invented by Navy Seal Randy Hetrick.

Twin Studies: Studies on paternal or identical twins designed to sort out environmental from genetic influences.

Type II Diabetes: Long term metabolic disorder characterized by high blood sugar, insulin resistance, and obesity. Classic symptoms include hunger, increased thirst, and increased urination. Long term complications include heart disease, stroke, retinopathy, neuropathy, blindness, kidney failure, impaired blood flow, and amputation.

Type III Diabetes: The condition of insulin resistance within the brain often related to Alzheimer's disease.

Vasoconstriction: Narrowing of the blood vessels resulting from contraction of muscular walls of the vessels resulting in increased blood pressure.

Vasopressin: A peptid hormone secreted by the adrenal gland causing water retention.

Victoza: The brand name for Liraglutide, glucagon-like peptic GLP-1 agonist medication. It is useful for weight loss and diabetes.

Visceral Fat: Fat deposits in the abdomen otherwise known as belly fat. This fat is active as an endocrine organ in secreting adipokines, hormones that can either harm or help health.

Visceral Obesity: The state where fat is stored primarily in the peritoneal cavity in-between organs that is strongly associated with insulin resistance, metabolic syndrome, and inflammatory and oxidative diseases such as cancer, cardiovascular disease, and dementia.

Vegan: Dietary practice of abstaining from the eating of animal products such as meat, egg, and cheese.

VLDL: Very low density lipoprotein manufactured by liver that can enhance transport of fats and cholesterols into cells. High levels are considered atherogenic.

VO2 Max: The highest rate of oxygen consumption during maximal exertion during aerobic activity.

Western Diet: A diet high in energy-dense food such as trans-fats, simple sugars, and saturated fats.

Whey Protein: A milk derived protein containing lactalbumin, lactoglobulin, lactoferrin, and immunoglobulins; the liquid portion of milk.

Western Life-Stye: Sedentary lifestyle with very little activity such as walking, standing, muscle contraction, or exercising of any sort is done.

White Coat Hypertension: Also known as white coat syndrome. A phenomenon where people exhibit blood pressure elevations clinically such as in the hospital or at their physician's office, but have normal pressure measurements at home. This was originally believed to be due to simple anxiety and it is now increasingly recognized to be associated with sympathetic hyperactivity associated with insulin resistance and metabolic syndrome.

Xanthine: Purine base found in most human tissues and fluids. A number of stimulants are derived from Xanthine including caffeine and theobromine.

Yoga: Physical activity consisting of postures, breathing exercises, and a period of relaxation or meditation.

REFERENCES

Chapter 1 References-The Metabolic Syndrome.

1. Lejeune, M., Kovacs, E., Westerterp-Plantenga, M. Additional protein intake limits weight regain after weight loss in humans. *British Journal of Nutrition.* 2005; 93(2): 281-289.

2. Melby, C., Scholl, C., Edwards, G., et al. Effects of acute resistance exercise on post exercise energy expenditure and resting metabolic rate. *Journal of Applied Physiology.* (1985). 1993; 75(4): 1847-53.

3. Sutton, E., Beyl, R., Early, K., et al. Early Time-Restricted Feeding Improves Insulin Sensitivity, Blood Pressure, and Oxidative Stress Even without Weight Loss in Men with Prediabetes. *Cell Metabolism.* 2018; 27(6): 1212-1221.

Chapter 2 References-Thrifty Genes, Skinny Genes

4. Zhang, Z., Zhang, R., Zhi-Zhen, Q., et al. Effects of Chronic Whey Protein Supplementation on Atherosclerosis in ApoE$^{-/-}$ Mice. *J. Nutr Science and Vitaminology.* 2018; 64(2): 143-150.

5. Tabung, F., Wang, W., Fung, T. et al. Development and validation of empirical indices to assess the insulinemic potential of diet and lifestyle. *Br. J. Nutr.* 2016; 8:1-12.

Chapter 3 References-The Coffee Cure Diet Plan

6. Akhavan, T., Luhovyy, B., Brown, P., et al. Effect of Premeal Consumption of Whey Protein and its Hydrolysate on Food Intake and Postmeal Glycemia and Insulin Responses in Young Adults. *American Journal of Clinical Nutrition.* 2010; 91(4): 966-75.

7. The Diabetes Prevention Program (DPP). *Diabetes Care.* 2002; 25(12): 2165-2171.

8. Karahalios, A., Simpson, J., Baglietto, L. et al. Changes in body size and mortality: results from the Melbourne collaborative cohort study. *PLoS One.* 2014; 10:1371.

9. Fraser, G., Shevlik, D. Ten Years of Life: Is It a Matter of Choice? *Arch Internal Medicine.* 2001; 161 (13): 1645-52.

10. Mignone, L., Wu, T., Horowitz, M., et al. Whey protein: The "whey" forward for the treatment of type 2 diabetes? *World J. Diabetes.* 2015; 6(14): 1274-84.

11. Tonstad, S., Stewart, K., Oda, K., et al. Vegetarian diets and incidence of diabetes in the Adventist Health Study-2. *Nutrition Metabolism and Cardiovascular Disease.* 2013; 23(4): 292-299.

12. Pal, S., Ellis, V., Ho, S. Acute effects of whey protein isolate on cardiovascular risk factors in overweight, post-menopausal women. *Atherosclerosis.* 2010; 2012(1): 339-44.

Chapter 4 References-Insulin Resistance: The Root of the Metabolic Syndrome

13. Kondo, T., Osugi, S., Shimokata, K., et al. Metabolic syndrome and all-cause mortality, cardiac events, and cardiovascular events: a follow-up study in 25,471 young and middle-aged Japanese men. *Eur J Cardiovasc Prev Rehabil.* 2011; 18(4): 574-80.

14. Mozaffarian, D., Katan, M., Ascherio, A., et al. Trans Fatty Acids and Cardiovascular Disease. *New England Journal of Medicine.* 2006; 354(15): 1601-13.

15. Helvaci, M., Kaya, H., Gundogdu, M. White coat hypertension may be an initial sign of metabolic syndrome. *Acta Med. Indones.* 2012; 44(3): 223-227.

16. Ferrannini, E., Haffner, S., Stern, M. Essential hypertension: An insulin-resistant state. *Journal of Cardiovascular Pharmacology.* 1990; 15 supplement 5:S18-25.

17. Defronzo, R., Ferrannini, E. Insulin resistance: A multifaceted syndrome responsible for NIDDM, obesity, hypertension, dyslipidemia, and atherosclerotic cardiovascular disease. *Diabetes Care.* 1991.

18. McCarty, M. A chlorogenic acid induced increase in GLP-1 production may mediate the impact of heavy coffee consumption on diabetes risk. *Med Hypotheses.* 2005; 64(4): 848-53.

19. Mignone, L., Wu, T., Horowitz, M., et al. Whey protein: The "whey" forward for the treatment of type 2 diabetes? *World J Diabetes.* 2015; 6(14): 1274-84.

20. Hutchison, A., Farrie-Bisset, C., Fitzgerald, P., et al. Comparative effects of intraduodenal whey protein hydrolysate on antropyloroduodenal motility gut hormones glycemia, appetite, and energy intake in lean and obese men. *Am J Clin Nutr* 2015; 102(6): 1323-31.

21. Lee, C., Yu, S., Kim, N., et al. Association between Coffee Consumption and Circulating Levels of Adiponectin and Leptin. *J Med Food.* 2017; 20(11): 1068-75.

22. Kim, K., Park, S. Association between the Prevalence of Metabolic Syndrome and the Level of Coffee Consumption among Korean Women. *PLoS One.* 2016; 11(12).

23. Gao, J., Song, J., Du, M., et al. Bovine ά-Lactalbumine Hydrosolate (ά-LAH) Ameliorates Adipose Insulin Resistance and Inflammation in High-Fat Diet-Fed C57BL/6J Mice. *Nutrients.* 2018; 10(2): 242.

24. Baspinar, B., Eskiol, G., Ozcelik, A., How coffee affects metabolic syndrome and its components. *Food Function.* 2017; 8(6): 2089-2101.

25. Sousa, G., Lira, F., Rosa, J., et al. Dietary whey protein lessens several risk factors for metabolic diseases: a review. *Lipids Health Disease.* 2012; July 10.

26. Chaix, A., Zarrinpar, A., Miu, P., et al. Time-restricted feeding is a preventative and therapeutic intervention against diffuse nutritional challenges. *Cell Metabo* 2014; 20(6): 991-1005.

27. Wood, J., O'Neal, E. Resistance Training in Type II Diabetes Mellitus: Impact on Areas of Metabolic Dysfunction in Skeletal Muscle and Potential Impact on Bone. *J Nutrition and Metabolism.* 2012; 268197.

Chapter 5 References-The Muscle Sink

28. Brooks, N., Layne, J., Gordon, P., et al. Strength training improves muscle quality and insulin sensitivity in Hispanic older adults with type 2 diabetes. *Int J Med Science.* 2006; 18; 4(1): 19-27.

29. Strasser, B., Pesta, D. Resistance Training for Diabetes Prevention and Therapy: Experimental Findings and Molecular Mechanisms. *Biomedical Research Int.* 2013; 805217.

30. Yang, Z, Scott, C, Mao, C., et al. Resistance exercise versus aerobic exercise for type 2 diabetes: a systematic review in meta-analysis. *Sports Medicine*: 2014; 44(4): 487-499.

31. Sinaki, M., Itoi, E., Wahner, H., et al. Stronger back muscles reduce the incidence of vertebral fractures: a prospective 10 year follow-up of postmenopausal women. *Bone.* 2002; 30(6): 836-841.

32. Ferrando, A., Tipton, K., Bamman, M., et al. Resistance exercise maintains skeletal muscle protein synthesis during bed rest. *J Appl. Physiol (1985).* 1997; 82(3): 807-810.

33. Kim, G., Lee, S., Jun, J., et al. Increase in relative skeletal muscle mass over time and its inverse association with metabolic syndrome development: A 7-year retrospective cohort study. *Cardiovascular Diabetology.* 2018; 17:23.

34. Seldin, M., Peterson, J., Byerly, M., et al. Myonectin (CTRP15), a novel myokine that links skeletal muscle to systemic lipid homeostasis. *J Biological Chemistry*. 2012; 287(15): 11968-11980.

35. Dominguez-Sanchez, M., Bustos-Cruz, R., Velasco-Orjuda, G., et al. Acute effects of high-intensity resistance, or combined protocol on the increase of the level of neurotrophic factors in physically inactive overweight adults: The BrainFit Study. *Front Physiol*. 2018; 9:741.

36. Tsukamoto, H., Suga, T., Takenaka, S., An acute bout of localized resistive exercise can rapidly improve inhibitor control. *PLoS-One*. 2017; 12(9): E0184075.

37. Fekete, A., Giromine, C., Chatzidiakou, Y., et al. Whey protein lowers blood pressure and improves endothelial function and lipid biomarkers in adults with prehypertension and mild hypertension: results from the chronic Whey2Go randomized control trial. *Am J Clin Nutr*. 2016; 104(6): 1534-1544.

38. Mehanna, H., Moledina, J., Travis, J., et al. Refeeding syndrome: what it is, and how to prevent and treat it. *BMJ*. 2008; 336(7659): 1495-1498.

39. Vandelbo, M., Clasen, B., Treebak, J., et al. Insulin resistance after a 72-hour fast is associated with impaired AS160 phosphorylation and accumulation of lipid and glycogen in human skeletal muscle. *Am J. Physiol Endocrinol Metab*. 2012; 302(2): E190-200.

40. Schwertzer, G., Arias, E., Cartee, G., Sustained post exercise increase in AS160 phosphorylation in skeletal muscle without sustained increase in kinase phosphorylation. *J Appl Physiol (1985)*. 2012: 113(12): 1852-1861.

41. Waters, D., Ward, A., Villareal, D., at al. Weight loss in obese adults 65-years and older: a review of the controversy. *Exp Gerontol*. 2013: 48(10): 1054-1061.

42. Voican, C., Lebrun, A., Maitre, S., et al. Predictive score of sarcopenia occurrence one year after bariatric surgery in severely obese patients. *PLoS One*. 2018; 13(5)E0197248.

43. Lu, C., Chang, Y., Chang, H., et al. Fracture Risk after Bariatric Surgery: A 12-Year National Cohort Study. *Medicine (Baltimore)*. 2014; 94(48)E2087.

Chapter 6 References-Your Body on the Coffee Cure

44. Ding, M., Satija, A., Bhupathiraju, S., et al. Association of Coffee Consumption with Total and Cause-Specific Mortality in 3 Large Prospective Cohorts. *Circ*. 2015; 132(24):2305-2315.

45. Van Dongen, L., Mölenberg, F., Soedamah-Muthu, S. et al. Coffee consumption after myocardial infarction and risk of cardiovascular mortality: a perspective analysis in the Alpha Omega Cohort. *Am J Clin Nutr.* 2017; 106(4): 1113-20.

46. Mukamal, K., Halqvist, J., Hammar, M., et al. Coffee consumption and mortality after a myocardial infarction: the Stockholm Heart Epidemiology Program. *Am Heart J.* 2009; 157(3): 495-501.

47. Brown, O., Allgar, V., Wong, K. Coffee reduces the risk of death after acute myocardial infarction: a meta-analysis. *Coran Artery Dis.* 2016; 27(7): 566-72.

48. Lecour, S., Lamont, K. Natural polyphenols and cardioprotection. *Mini Rev Med Chem.* 2011; 11(14): 1191-9.

49. Klatsky, A., Hasan, A., Armstrong, M., et al. Coffee, caffeine, and risk of hospitalization for arrhythmias. *Perm J.* 2011; 15(3): 19-25.

50. Pirillo, A., Norata, G., Catapano, A., Postprandial lipemia as a cardiometabolic risk factor. *Curr Med Res Opin.* 2014; 30(8): 1489-503.

51. Stanstrup, J., Schou, S., Holmer-Jensen, J., et al. Whey protein delays gastric emptying and suppresses plasma fatty acids and their metabolites compared to casein, gluten, and fish protein. *J. Proteome Res.* 2014; 13(5): 2301-2408.

52. Pal, S., Ellis, V., Ho, S., Acute effects of whey protein isolate on cardiovascular risk factors in overweight, postmenopausal women. *Atherosclerosis.* 2010; 212(1): 339-344.

53. Ding, M., Bhupathirju, S., Chen, M., et al. Caffeinated and decaffeinated coffee consumption and risk of type 2 diabetes: a systemic review and a dose-response meta-analysis. *Diabetes Care.* 2014; 37(2): 569-86.

54. Yarmolinsky, J., Mueller, N., Duncan, B., et al. Coffee Consumption, Newly Diagnosed Diabetes, and Other Alterations in Glucose Homeostasis: A Cross-Sectional Analysis of the Longitudinal Study of Adult Health. (ELSA-Brasil) *PLoS One.* 2015.

55. McCarty, M. A chlorogenic acid-induced increase in GLP-1 production may mediate the impact of heavy coffee consumption on diabetes risk. *Med Hypotheses.* 2005; 64(4): 848-53.

56. Mignone, L., Wu, T., Horowitz, M., et al. Whey protein: The "whey" forward for the treatment of type 2 diabetes? *World J. Diabetes.* 2015; 6 (14): 1274-84.

57. Sutton, E., et al. Early Time-Restricted Feeding Improves Insulin Sensitivity, Blood Pressure, and Oxidative Stress even without Weight Loss in Men with Prediabetes. *Cell Metabolism*. 2018; 27(6): 1212-1221.

58. Carrieri, M., Protopopescu, C., Marcellin, F., et al. Protective effect of coffee consumption on all-cause mortality of French HIV-HCV co-infected patients. *J. Hepatol*. 2017; 67(6):1157-1167.

59. Freedman, N., Everhart, J., Lindsay, K., et al. Coffee intake is associated with lower rates of liver disease progression in chronic hepatitis C. *Hepatology*. 2009; 50(5):1360-1369.

60. Lai, G., Weinstein, S., Albanes, D., et al. The association of coffee intake with liver cancer incidence and chronic liver disease mortality in male smokers. *Br J. Cancer*. 2013;109(5):1344-1351.

61. Morifuji, M., Sakai, K., Sanbongi, C., et al. Dietary whey protein downregulates fatty acid synthesis in the liver, but upregulates it in skeletal muscle of exercise-trained rats. *Nutrition*. 2005; 21(10):1052-1058.

62. Bortolotti, M., Maiolo, E., Corazza, M., et al. Effects of a whey protein supplementation on intrahepatocellular lipids in obese female patients. *Clin Nutr*. 2011; 30(4):494-498.

63. Kume, H., Okazaki, K., Sasaki, AH. Hepatoprotective effects of whey protein on D-galactosamine-induced hepatitis and liver fibrosis in rats. *Biosci Biotechnol Biochem*. 2006; 70(5):1281-1285.

64. Chaix, A., Zarrinpar, A., Miu, P., et al. Time-Restrictive Feeding Is a Preventative and Therapeutic Intervention against Diverse Nutritional Challenges. *Cell Metabo* 2014; 20(6): 991-1005.

65. Berenbaum, F. Osteoarthritis as an inflammatory disease. *Osteoarthritis Cartilage*. 2013; 21(1): 16-21.

66. Chauhan, S., Satti, N., Sharma, V., et al. Amelioration of inflammatory responses by Chlorogenic acid via suppression of pro-inflammatory mediators. *Journal of Applied Science*. 2011; 01(04): 67-75.

67. Liang, N., Kitts, D., Role of Chlorogenic Acids in Controlling Oxidative and Inflammatory Stress Conditions. *Nutrients*. 2016; 8(1): 16.

68. Zhou, L., Xu, J., Han, S., et al. Effect of whey supplementation on circulating C-reactive protein: a meta-analysis of randomized controlled trials. *Nutrients*. 2015; 7(2): 1131-1143.

69. Morro, T. Tinsley, G., Bianco, A., et al. Effects of eight-weeks of time-restricted feeding (16/8) on basal metabolism, maximal strength, body composition, inflammation, and cardiovascular risk factors in resistance-trained males. *J Transl Med.* 2016; 14: 290.

70. Jacob, T., Benowitz, N., Destaillats, H., et al. Thirdhand Smoke: New Evidence, Challenges, and Future Directions. *Chem Res Toxicol.* 2017; 30(1): 270-94.

71. Fukai, T., Ushio-Fukai, M. Superoxide dismutases: role in redox signaling, vascular function, and diseases. *Antiox Redox Signal.* 2011; 15(6): 1583-1606.

72. Liu, Y., Hyde, A., Simpson, M., et al. Emerging regulatory paradigms in glutathione metabolism. *Adv Cancer Res.* 2014; 122(69-101).

73. Doganay, S., Turaoz, Y., Evereklioglu, C., et al. Use of caffeic acid phenethyl ester to prevent sodium-selenite-induced cataract in rat eyes. *J Cataract Refract Surg.* 2002; 28(8): 1457-62.

74. Varma, S. Effect of coffee (caffeine) against human cataract blindness. *Clin Ophthalmol* 2016; 10:213-220.

75. Je, Y., Giovannucci, E. Coffee consumption and total mortality: a meta-analysis of twenty prospective cohort studies. *Br J Nutr.* 2014; 111(7): 1162-73.

76. Poole, R., Kennedy, O., Roderick, P., et al. Coffee consumption and health: umbrella review of meta-analysis of multiple health outcomes. *BMJ.* 2017; 359:5024.

77. Grosso, G., Godos, J., Galvano, F., et al. Coffee, Caffeine, and Health Outcomes: An Umbrella Review. *Annu Rev Nutr.* 2017; 37:131-156.

78. Kent, K., Harper, W., Bomser, J. Effect of whey protein isolate on intracellular glutathione and oxidant-induced cell death in human prostate epithelial cells. *Toxicol In Vitro.* 2003; 17(1): 27-33.

79. Kita, M., Kobayashi, K., Obara, K., et al. Supplementation With Whey Peptide Rich in ß-Lactolin Improves Cognitive Performance in Healthy Older Adults: A Randomized Double-Blind Placebo-Controlled Study. *Front. Neurosci.* 2019; 13:399.

80. Lejeune, M., Kovacs, E., Westerterp-Plantega, M. Additional protein intake limits weight regain after weight loss in humans. *British Journal of Nutrition.* 2005; 93(2): 261-9.

81. Lucas, M., O'Reilly, E., Pan, A., et al. Coffee, caffeine, and risk of completed suicide: results from three perspective cohorts of American adults. *World J. Biol Psychiatry.* 2014; 15(5): 377-86.

82. Klatsky, A, Armstrong, M., Friedman, G., Coffee, tea, and mortality. *Ann Epidemiol.* 1993; 3(4): 375-81.

83. Kawachi, L., Willett, W., Colditz, G., et al. A prospective study of coffee drinking and suicide in women. *Arch Intern Med.* 1996; 156(5): 521-25.

84. Ruusunen, A., Lehto, S., Tolmunen, T., et al. Coffee, tea, and caffeine intake and the risk of severe depression in middle-aged Finnish men: the Kuopio Ischaemia Heart Disease Risk Factor Study. *Public Health Nutrition.* 2010; 13(8): 1215-20.

85. Geleijnse, J. Habitual coffee consumption and blood pressure: an epidemiological perspective. *Vasc Health Risk Manag.* 2008;4(5):963-970.

86. Xie, C., Cui, L., Zhu, J., et al. Coffee consumption and risk of hypertension: A systematic review and dose-response meta-analysis of cohort studies. *J Hum Hypertens.* 2018;32(2): 83-93.

87. Chrysant, S., Chrysant, G. Cardiovascular complications from consumption of high energy drinks: recent evidence. *J Hum Hypertens* 2015: 29(2):71-76.

88. Dineley, K., Jahrling, J., Denner, L., et al. Insulin resistance in Alzheimer's disease *Neurobiol Dis* 2014.

89. Ng, T., Feng, L., Niti, M., et al. Can coffee consumption lower risk of Alzheimer's disease? *JAMA* 2016; 34(4): 941-953.

90. Soffrizzi, V., Scafato, E., Capurso, C., et al. Metabolic syndrome and the risk of vascular dementia: The Italian Longitudinal Study on Ageing. *J Neurol Neurosurg Psychiatry.* 2010; 81: 1433-440.

91. Eskelinen, M., Nguandu, T., Tuomilehto, J., et al. Midlife coffee and tea drinking and the risk of late-life dementia; a population-based CAIDE study. *J Alzheimers Dis.* 2009; 16(1):

85-91.

92. Arendash, G., Mori, T., Cao, C., et al. Caffeine reverses cognitive impairment and decreases brain amyloid-beta levels in aged Alzheimer's disease mice. *J Alzheimers Dis.* 2009; 17(3): 661-80.

93. Vangelder, B., Buijssee, B., Tijhuis, M., et al. Coffee consumption is inversely associated with cognitive decline in elderly European men: The FINE Study. *EUR J Clin Nutr.* 2007; 61(2): 226-32.

94. Ritchie, K., Carriére, I., Mendonca, A., et al. Neuroprotective effects of caffeine: a prospective population study (The Three City Study). *Neurology.* 2007; 69(6): 536-45.

95. Barranco-Quintana, J., Allam, M., Serrano-del Castillo, A., et al. Alzheimer's disease and coffee: a quantitative review. *Neurol Res.* 2007; 29(1): 91-95.

96. Lopez-Garcia, E., Rodriguez-Artalejo, F., Rexroad, K., et al. Coffee consumption and risk of stroke in women. *Circulation.* 2009; 119(8): 1116-23.

97. Lee, J., Lee, J., Kim, Y. Relationship between coffee consumption and stroke risk in Korean population: the Health Examinees (HEXA Study). *Nutr J.* 2017; 16(7).

98. Mineharu, Y., Koizumi, A., Wada, Y., et al. Coffee, green tea, black tea, and oolong tea consumption and risk of mortality from cardiovascular disease in Japanese men and women. *J Epidemiol Community Health* 2011; 65(3): 230-40.

99. Kita, M. Obara, K., Kondo, S., et al. Effect of Supplementation of Whey Peptide. *Nutrients.* 2018; 10(7): 899.

100. Shertzer, H., Krishan, M., Genter, M., et al. Dietary whey protein stimulates mitochondrial activity and decreases oxidative stress in mouse female brain. *Neuroscience letter.* 2013; 548:159-164.

101. Journel, M., Chaumontet, C., Darcel, N., et al. Brain responses to high protein diets. *Advances in Nutrition.* 2012; 3(3): 322-329.

102. Maciejczyk, M., Zebrowska, E., Chabowski, A. Insulin Resistance and Oxidative Stress in the Brain: What is New? *Int J Mol. Sci.* 2019; 20(4): 874.

103. Bae, C., Song, J. The Role of Glucagon-Like Peptid I (GLP-1) in Type 3 Diabetes: GLP-1 Controls Insulin Resistance, Neuroinflammation, and Neurogenesis in the Brain. *Int J Mol Sci.* 2017; 18(11): 2493.

104. Sabir, S, Saleen, A., Akhtar, M., et al. Increasing beta cell mass to treat diabetes mellitus. *Adv Clin Exp Med.* 2018; 27(9):1309-1315.

105. Nakamura, K., Haglind, E., Achenbach, S., et al. Fracture risk following bariatric surgery: a population-based study. *Osteoporos Int.* 2014; 25(1): 151-158.

106. Gabal, K., Hoddy, K., Haggerty, N., et al. Effects of eight-hour time restrictive feeding on body weight and metabolic disease risk factors in obese adults: A pilot study. *Nutr. Healthy Aging.* 2018; 4(4): 345-353.

107. Choi, E., Choi, K., Park, S., et al. The Benefit of Bone Health by Drinking Coffee among Korean Postmenopausal Women: A Cross Sectional-Analysis of the Fourth & Fifth Korea National Health and Nutrition Examination Surveys. *PLoS One.* 2016.

108. Underwood, P., Adler, G. The renin angiotensin aldosterone system and insulin resistance in humans. *Current Hypertension Reviews.* 2013; 15(1): 59-70.

109. Fekete, A., Giromine, C., Chatzidiakou, Y., et al. Whey protein lowers blood pressure and improves endothelial function and lipid biomarkers in adults with prehypertension and mild hypertension: results from the chronic Whey2Go randomized control trial. *Am J Clin Nutr.* 2016; 104(6): 1534-1544.

110. Tyson, C., Nwankwo, C., Lin, P., et al. The Dietary Approaches to Stop Hypertension (DASH) eating pattern in special populations. *Curr Hypertens Rep.* 2012; 14(5): 388-396.

111. Bhullar, K., et al. Antihypertensive effect of caffeic acid and its analogs through its dual renin-angiotensin-aldosterone system inhibition. *Eur J. Pharmacol.* 2014.

112. Nie, J., et al. Caffeic acid phenethyl esters ameliorate insulin resistance by inhibiting JNK and NFKB inflammatory pathways in diabetic mice and Hep G2 cell modules. *J Agricul Food Chem.* 2017.

113. Watanabe, H., Tanabe, N., Watanabe, T., et al. Metabolic studies and risk of development of atrial fibrillation. *Circulation.* 2008; 117(10): 1255-1260.

114. Lubbers, E., Price, M., Mohler, P., Arrhythmogenic Substrates for Atrial Fibrillation in Obesity. *Front Physiol.* 2018; Oct 22; 9:1482.

115. Seccia, T., Caroccia, B., Adler, G., et al. Arterial Hypertension, Atrial Fibrillation, and Hyperaldosteronism: The Triple Trouble. *Hypertension.* 2017; 69(4): 545-550.

116. Loftfield, E., Freedman, N., Graubard, B., et al. Coffee drinking and cutaneous melanoma risk in the NIH-AARP diet and health study. *J Natl Cancer Inst.* 2015; 107(2): DJU421.

117. Caini, S., Masala, G., Saieva, C., et al. Coffee, tea and melanoma risk: findings from the European Prospective Investigation into Cancer and Nutrition. *Int J Cancer.* 2017; 140(10): 2246-2255.

118. Song, F., Qureshi, A., Han, J. Increased caffeine intake is associated with reduced risk of basal call carcinoma of the skin. *Cancer Res.* 2012; 72(13): 3282-3289.

119. Fukushima, Y., Takahashi, Y., Hori, Y., et al. Skin photprotection and consumption of coffee and polyphenols in healthy middle-aged Japanese females. *Int J Dermatol.* 2015; 54(4): 410-418.

120. Cho, Y., Bahuguna, A., Kim, H., et al. Potential effect of compounds isolated from Coffea arabica against UV-B induced skin damage by protecting fibroblast cells. *J Photochem Photobiol B*. 2017; 174:323-332.

121. Cani, P., Amar, J., Iglesias, M., et al. Metabolic Endotoxemia Initiates Obesity and Insulin Resistance. *Diabetes*. 2007; 57(7): 1761-1772.)

122. Lee, C. The Effect of High-Fat Diet-Induced Pathophysiological Changes in the Gut on Obesity: What Should be the Ideal Treatment? *Clin Transl Gastroenterol*. 2013 11;4: E39.

123. Sanmiguel C., Gupta, A, Mayer, E. Gut Microbiome and Obesity: A Plausible Explanation for Obesity. *Curr Obes Rep*. 2015; 4(2): 250-261.

124. Choi, J., Park, S., Jung, J., et al. Caffeic Acid Cyclohexylamide Rescues Lethal Inflammation in Septic Mice through Inhabitation of 1κB Kinase in Innate Immune Process. *Sci Rep*. 2017; 7: 41180.

125. Ruan, Z., Liu, S., Zhou, Y., et al. Chlorogenic acid decreases intestinal permeability and increases expression of intestinal tight junction proteins in weaned rats challenged with LPS. *PLoS One*. 2014; 9(6): E97815.

126. Xiao, K, Jiao, L, Cao, S., et al. Whey protein concentrate enhances intestinal integrity and influences transforming growth factor-ß1 and mitogen-activated protein kinase signaling pathways in piglets after lipopolysaccharide challenge. *Br J. Nutr*. 2016; 115(6): 984-93.

127. Causey, J., Thompson, K. The way to intestinal health.

128. Kell, D., Pretorius, E. On the translocation of bacteria and lipopolysaccharides between blood and peripheral locations in chronic inflammatory diseases: the central roles of LPS and LPS-induced cell death. *Integr. Biol (Camb)*. 2015; 7(11):1339-1377.

129. Vasconcelos, A., Yshii, L., Viel, T., et al. Intermittent fasting attenuates lipopolysaccharide-induced neuroinflammation and memory impairment. *J. Neuroinflammation*. 2014; 11:85.

130. Phillips, M., Flynn, M., McFarlin, B, et al. Resistive exercise blunts LPS-stimulated TNF-ἁ and I1-Iß. *Int J. Sports Med* 2008; 29(2): 102-9.

131. Glick-Bauer, M. Yeh, M. The health advantage of a vegan diet: exploring the gut microbiota connection. *Nutrients*. 2014; 31; 6(11): 4822-4838.

132. Banks, W., Farr, S., Salameh, T. et al. Triglycerides cross the blood-brain barrier and induce central leptin and insulin receptor resistance. *Int J Obes. (Lond)*. 2018; 42(3): 391-397.

133. Vercambre, M., Berr, C., Ritchie, K., et al. Caffeine and cognitive decline in elderly women at vascular risk. *J Alzheimers Dis.* 2013; 35(2): 10.3233.

134. Ullah, F., Ali, T., Ullah, N., et al. Caffeine prevents d-galactose induced cognitive deficits, oxidative stress, neuroinflammation, and neurodegeneration in the adult rat brain. *Neurochem Int* 2015; 90: 114-24.

135. Arendash, G., Mori, T., Koco, C., et al. Caffeine reverses cognitive impairment and decreases brain amyloid-beta levels in aged Alzheimer's disease mice. *J Alzheimer's Dis.* 2009; 17 (3):661-680.

136. Lopez-Cruz, L., Salamone, J., Correa, M. The Impact of Caffeine on the Behaviorial Effects of Ethenol Related to Abuse and Addiction: A Review of Animal Studies. *J. Caffeine Res.* 2013; 3(1): 9-21.

137. Shukitt-Hale, B., Miller, M., Chu, Y., et al. Coffee, but not caffeine, has positive effects on cognition and psychomotor behavior in aging. *Age (Dordr).* 2013; 35(6): 2183-2192.

138. Felger, J., Lotrich, F. Inflammatory cytokines in depression: neurobiological mechanisms and therapeutic implications. *Neuroscience.* 2013; 246:199-229.

139. Zhang, J., Yue, Y., Thapa, A., et al. Baseline serum C-reactive protein levels may predict antidepressant treatment responses in patients with major depressive disorder. *J Affect Disord.* 2019; 250: 432-438.

140. Osimo, E., Cardinal, R., Jones, P., et al. Prevalence and correlates of low-grade systemic inflammation in adult psychiatric inpatients: An electronic health record-based study. *Psychoneuroendocrinology.* 2018; 91: 226-234.

141. Köhler, O., Krogh, J., Mors, O., et al. Inflammation In Depression and Potential for Anti-Inflammatory Treatment. *Curr Neuropharmicol.* 2016; 14(7): 732-742.

142. Li, Y, Zhong, X., Cheng, G., et al. Hs-CRP and all-cause, cardiovascular, and cancer mortality risk: a meta-analysis. *Atherosclerosis.* 2017: 259:75-82.

143. Eraly, S., Nievergelt, C., Maihofer, A., et al. Assessment of plasma C-reactive protein as a biomarker of posttraumatic stress disorder risk. *JAMA Psychiatry.* 2014; 71(4): 423-31.

144. Suarez, E., Sundy, J. The cortisol: C-reactive protein ratio and negative affect reactivity in depressed adults. *Health Psychol.* 2017; 36(9): 852-862.

145. Nowakowski, A. Chronic inflammation and quality of life in older adults: A cross-sectional study using biomarkers to predict emotional and relational outcomes. *Health Qual Life Outcomes.* 2014; 12:141.

146. Dinh, K., Kaspersen, K., Mikkelsen, S., et al. Low-grade inflammation is negatively associated with physical Health-Related Quality of Life in healthy individuals: Results from the Danish Blood Donor Study (DBDS). *PLoS One.* 2019; 14(3): E0214468.

147. Ho, K., Lipman, J. An update on C-reactive protein for intensivists. *Anesth Intensive Care.* 2009; 37(2): 234-41.

148. Sbarra, D. Marriage protects men from clinically meaningful elevations in C-reactive protein: results from the National Social Life Health in Aging Project. (NSHAP). *Psychosom Med.* 2009; 71(8): 828-35.

149. Lacey, R., Kumari, M., McMunn, A. Parenteral separation in childhood and adult inflammation: the importance of material and psychosocial pathways. *Psychoneuroendocrinology.* 2013; 38(11): 2476-84.

150. Nikulina, V. Do race, neglect, and childhood poverty predict physical health in adulthood? A multilevel perspective analysis. *Child Abuse Negl.* 2014; 38(3): 414-424.

151. Newton, T., Fernandez-Botran, R., Miller, J., et al. Markers of Inflammation in Midlife Women with Intimate Partner Violence Histories. *J Womens Health (Larchmt).* 2011; 20(12):1871-1880.

152. Boch, S., Ford, J. C-Reactive Protein Levels Among U.S. adults Exposed to Parenteral Incarceration. *Biol Res Nurs.* 2014; 17(5):574-584.

153. Oishi, J., Castro, C., Silva, K., et al. Endothelial Dysfunction and Inflammation Precedes Elevations in Blood Pressure Induced by a High-Fat Diet. *Arg Bras Cardiol.* 2018; 110(6): 558-567.

154. Bettcher, B., Wilheim, R, Rigby, T., et al. C-reactive protein is related to memory and medial temporal brain volume in older adults. *Brain Behav Immun.* 2012; 26(1): 103-108.

155. Hang, D., Kvaerner, A., Ma, W., et al. Coffee consumption and plasma biomarkers of metabolic and inflammatory pathways in U.S. health professionals. *Am J Clin Nutr.* 2019; 109(3):635-647.

156. Zhou, L., Xu, J., Rao, C. et al. Effect of whey supplementation on circulating C-reactive protein: a meta-analysis of randomized controlled trials. *Nutrients.* 2015; 7(2): 1131-43.

157. Takeuchi, T., Matsunaga, K., Sugiyama, A. Antidepressant-like effect of milk-derived lactoferrin in the repeated forced-swim stress mouse model. *J Vet Med Sci* 2017; 79(11):1803-1806.

158. Mattson, N., Longo, V., Harvie, M. Impact of intermittent fasting on health and disease processes. *Ageing Res Rev.* 2017; 39:46-58.

159. Adams, A., Wirth, M., Khan, S., et al. The association of C-reactive protein and physical activity among a church-based population of African Americans. *Prev Med.* 2015; 77:137-40.

160. Ironson, G., Lucette, A., Hylton, E., et al. The Relationship Between Religious and Psychospiritual Measures and an Inflammatory Marker (CRP) in older Adults Experiencing Life Event Stress. *J. Relig Health.* 2018; 57(4): 1554-1566.

161. Bower, J., Irwin, M. Mind-body therapies and control of inflammatory biology: A descriptive review. *Brain Behav Immun.* 2016; 51:1-11.

162. Haghighatdoost, F., Bellissimo, N., Zepetnek, J. Association of vegetarian diet with inflammatory biomarkers: a systematic review and meta-analysis of observational studies. *Public Health Nutr.* 2017; 20(15): 2713-2721.

163. Nettleton, J., Follis, J., Schabath, M. Coffee intake, smoking, and pulmonary function in the Atherosclerosis Risk in Communities Study. *AM J Epidemiol* 2009; 169 (12): 1445-1453.

164. Pagano, R., Negri, E., Decarli, A., et al. Coffee drinking and prevalence of bronchial asthma. *Chest.* 1988:94 (2): 386-9.

165. Sugawara, K., Takahashi, H., Kasai, C., et al. Effects of nutritional supplementation combined with low-intensity exercise in malnourished patients with COPD. *Respir Med.* 2010; 104:1883-1889.

166. Leuzzi, G., Galeone, C., Taverna, F., et al. C-reactive protein levels predict mortality in COPD: a systemic review and meta-analysis. *European Respiratory Review.* 2017; 31;26(143): 160070.

167. Mann, S., Connett, J., Anthonisen, N., et al. C-reactive protein and mortality in mild to moderate chronic obstructive pulmonary disease. *Thorax.* 2006;61 (10): 849-853.

168. Sugawara, K., Takahashi, H., Kashiwagura, T., et al. Effective of anti-inflammatory supplementation with whey peptide and exercise therapy in patients with COPD. *Respiratory Medicine* 2012; 106:1526-1534.

169. Sonoda, N., Morimoto, A., Tatsumi, Y. et al. A prospective study of the impact of diabetes mellitus on restrictive and obstructive lung function impairment: The Saku Study. *Metabolism.* 2018; 82:58-64.

170. Hang, D., Kavaerner, A., Ma, W., et al. Coffee consumption and plasma biomarkers of metabolic and inflammatory pathways in U.S. health professionals. *AM J Clin. Nutr.* 2019; 109(3) 635-647.

171. Polkey, M., Moxham, J. Attacking the disease spiral in chronic obstructive pulmonary disease. *Clin Med.* (Lond). 2006; 6 (2) 190-196.

172. McDonald, V., Gibson, P., Scott, H. et al. Should we treat obesity in COPD? The effects of diet and resistive exercise training. *Respirology.* 2016; 21 (5): 875-82.

173. Kishta, O., Iskandar, M., Dauletbaev, N., et al. Pressurized whey protein can limit bacterial burden and protein oxidation in pseudomonas aeruginosa Lung Infection. *Nutrition.* 2013; 29 (6): 918-24.

174. Marshall, L., Oguejiofor, W., Price, R., et al. Investigation of the enhanced antimicrobial activity of combination dry powder inhaler formulations of lactoferrin. *Int. J. Pharm.* 2016; 514 (2): 399-406.

175. Valenti, P., Catizone, A., Pantanella, F., et al. Lactoferrin decreases inflammatory response by cystic fibrosis bronchial cells invaded with Burkholderia cenocepacia iron-Modulated Biofilm. *Int. J. Immunopathol. Pharmacol.* 2011: 24 (4): 1057-68.

176. Lands, L., Iskandar, M., Beaudoin, N., et al. Dietary supplementation with pressurized whey in patients with cystic fibrosis. *J. Med. Food.* 2010: 13 (1): 77-82.

177. Grey, V., Mohammed, S., Smountas, A., et al. Improved glutathione status in young adult patients with cystic fibrosis supplemented with whey protein. *J. Cyst. Fibros.* 2013; (4): 195-198.

178. Wakabayashi, H., Oda, H., Yamauchi, K., et al. Lactoferrin for prevention of common viral infections. *J. Infect. Chemother.* 2014; 20 (11): 666-71.

179. Vitetta, L., Coulson, S., Beck, S., et al. The clinical efficacy of a bovine lactoferrin/whey protein Ig-rich fraction (Lf/IgF) for the common cold: A double-blind randomized study. *Complement Ther Med* 2013; 21(3):164-71.

180. Karsch-Völk, M., Barrett, B., Linde, K. Echinacea for preventing and treating the common cold. *Jamma.* 2015; 313 (6): 618-9.

181. LeGrand, D. Lactoferrin, a Key Molecule in Immune and Inflammatory Processes. *Biochem. Cell Biol.* 2012; 90 (3): 252-68.

182. Reading, J., Meyers, A., Vyakarnam, A. Whey acidic proteins (WAPs): novel modulators of innate immunity to HIV infection. *Curr. Opin. HIV. AIDS.* 2012; 7 (2): 172-179.

183. Alfaro, T., Monteiro, R., Cunha, R., et al. Chronic coffee consumption and respiratory disease: A systematic review. *Clin. Respir. J.* 2018; 12 (3): 1283-1294.

Chapter 7 References-All Diets Are Not Created Equal

184. Kromhout, D., Keys, A., Aravanis, C., et al. Food consumption patterns in the 1960s in seven countries. *Am J Clin Nutr.* 1989; 49(5): 889-94.

185. Lauretti, E, Iuliano, L., Pratico, D., et al. Extra-virgin olive oil ameliorates cognition and neuropathology of the 3xTg mice: role of autophagy. *Ann Clin Transl Neurol_*2017; 4(8):564-574.

186. Lauretti, E, Pratico, D. Effect of canola oil consumption on memory, synapse, and neuropathology in the triple transgenic mouse model of Alzheimer's disease. *Sci Rep* 2017; 7:17134.

187. Coconut oil and dementia. Alzheimer's Society; united against dementia. Retrieved from www.Alzheimer's .org.UK.

188. Mori, T., Vandongen, R., Masarei, J., et al. Comparison of diets supplemented with fish oil or olive oil on plasma lipoproteins in insulin-dependent diabetics. *Metabolism.* 1991; 40(3): 241-246.

189. Medina-Remón, A., Casas, R., Tressserra-Rimbau, A., et al. Polyphenol intake from a Mediterranean diet decreases inflammatory biomarkers related to atherosclerosis: a sub-study of the PREDIMED trial. *Br J Clin Pharmacol.* 2017; 83(1):114-128.

190. Soriguer, F., Rojo-Martinez, G., Dobarganes, M., et al. Hypertension is related to the degradation of dietary frying oils. *Am J Clin Nutr.* 2003; 78(6):1092-7.

191. Srivastava, S., Singh, M., George, J., et al. Genotoxic and carcinogenic risks associated with the dietary consumption of repeatedly heated coconut oil. *Br J Nutr.* 2010; 104(9):1343-52.

192. Ayari, D., Boukazoula, F., Soumati, B., et al. Evaluation of oxidative stress biomarkers of rabbits' liver exposed to thermooxidized virgin olive oil obtained from blanquette olive cultivars. *Biomarkers.* 2019; 25:1-7.

193. Casal, S., Malheiro, R., Sendas, A., et al. Olive oil stability under deep-frying conditions. *Food Chem Toxicol.* 2010; 48(10):2972-9.

194. Mozaffarian, D., Katan, M., Ascherio, A., et al. Trans Fatty Acids and Cardiovascular Disease. *New England Journal of Medicine.* 2006; 354(15):1601-13.

195. Dobarganes, C., Marquez-Ruiz, G. Possible adverse effects of frying with vegetable oils. *Br J Nutr.* 2015; 113 Suppl 2:S49-57.

196. Ng, C., Leong, X., Masbah, N., et al. Heated vegetable oils and cardiovascular disease risk factors. *Vasul Pharmacol.* 2014; 61(1):1-9.

197. Qi, Q, Chu, A., Kang, J., et al. Fried food consumption, genetic risk, and body mass index: gene-diet interaction analysis in three U.S. cohort studies. *BMJ* 2014; 348:G1610.

198. Vormund, K., Braun, J., Rohrmann, S., et al. Mediterranean diet and mortality in Switzerland: an alpine paradox? *Eur J Nutr.* 2015; 54(1):139-48.

199. Hoffman, J. Protein—which is best? *J Sports Sci Med.* 2004; 3(3):118-130.

200. Sattar, N., Gaw, A., Scherbakova, O., et al. Metabolic syndrome with and without C- reactive protein as a predictor of coronary heart disease and diabetes in The West of Scotland Coronary Prevention Study. *Circulation.* 2003; 108(4):414-419.

201. Lee, C., Liese, A., Wagenknecht, L., et al. Fish consumption, insulin sensitivity and beta-cell function in the Insulin-resistant Atherosclerosis Studies (IRAS). *Nutr Metab Cardiovasc Dis.* 2013; 23(9): 829-835.

202. Orlich, M., Fraser, G. Vegetarian diet in the Adventist Health Study 2: A review of initial published findings. *Am J Clin Nutr.* 2014; 100(1): 353S-358S.

203. Zhang, J., Kesteloot, H. Differences in all-cause, cardiovascular and cancer mortality between Hong King and Singapore: role of nutrition. *Eur J Epidemiol.* 2001; 17(5): 469-477.

204. Reaven, G. Why syndrome X? From Harold Himsworth to the insulin resistance syndrome (IRS). *Cell Metabolism.* 2005; 1(1); 9-14.

205. Ruidavets, J., Bongard, V., Dallongeville, J., et al. High consumptions of grain, fish, dairy products, and combinations of these are associated with a low prevalence of metabolic syndrome. *J Epidemiol Community Health.* 2007; 61(9): 810-817.

206. Phillips, R., Garfinkel, L., Kuzma, J., et al. Mortality among California Seventh-Day Adventists for selected cancer sites. *J Natl Cancer Inst.* 1980; 65(5): 1097-1107.

207. Beeson, W., Mills, P., Phillips R., et al. Chronic disease among Seventh-Day Adventists, a low-risk group: Rationale, methodology, and description of the population. *Cancer.* 1989; 64(3): 570-581.

208. Fraser, G., Shavlik, D. Ten years of life: Is it a matter of choice? *Arch Intern Med.* 2001; 161(13): 1645-1652.

209. Orlich, M., Sing, P., Sabaté, J., et al. Vegetarian dietary patterns and mortality in Adventists Health Study II. *JAMA intern med.* 2013; 173(13): 1230-1238.

210. Hirayama, T. Mortality in Japanese with life-styles similar to Seventh-Day Adventists: strategy for risk reduction by life-style modification. *Natl Cancer Inst. Monogr.* 1985; 69: 143-153.

211. Giem, P., Beeson, W., Fraser, G. The Incidence of Dementia and Intake of Animal Products: Preliminary Findings from the Adventists Health Study. *Neuroepidemiology.* 1993; 12(1): 28-36.

212. Phillips, R., Lemon, F., Beeson, W., at al. Coronary heart disease mortality among Seventh-Day Adventists with differing dietary habits: a preliminary report. *AM J. Clin Nutr.* 1978; 31(10): S191-S198.

213. Stefler, D., Malyutina, S., Kubinova, R., et al. Mediterranean diet score and total cardiovascular mortality in Eastern Europe: the HAPIEE study. *Eur J. Nutri.* 2017; 56(1): 421-429.

214. Estruch, R., Martinez-Gonzalez, M., Corella-D., et al. Effects of a Mediterranean-style diet on cardiovascular risk factors: a randomized trial. *Ann Intern Med.* 2006; 145(1):1-11.

215. Vormund K., Braun, J., Rohrmann, S., et al. Mediterranean diet and mortality in Switzerland: an alpine paradox? *Eur J Nutr.* 2015; 54(1):139-148.)

216. Lordan, R., Zabetakis, L. Invited review: The anti-inflammatory properties of dairy lipids. *Journal of Dairy Science.* 2017; 100(6):4197-4212.

217. (Lordan, R., Tsoupras, A., Mitra, B., et al. Dairy Fats and Cardiovascular Disease: Do We Really Need to be Concerned? *Foods.* 2018; 7(3):29.

218. Panagiotakos, D., Pitsavos, C., Zampelas, A., et al. Dairy products consumption is associated with decreased levels of inflammatory markers related to cardiovascular disease in apparently healthy adults: the ATTICA study. *J Am Coll Nutr.* 2010; 29(4):357-364.

219. Stancliffe, A., Thorpe, T., Zemel, M. Dairy attenuates oxidative and inflammatory stress in metabolic syndrome. *Am J Clin Nutr.* 2011; 94(2):422-30.

Chapter 8 References-Coffee Cure Tips and Tactics

220. Marinac, C., Nelson, S., Breen, C. Prolonged Nightly Fasting and Breast Cancer prognosis. *JAMA Oncol.* 2016; 2(8): 1049-1055.

221. Emerson, S., Kurti, S., Harms, C., et al. Magnitude and Timing of the Postprandial Inflammatory Response to a High-Fat Meal in Healthy Adults: A Systematic Review. *Adv. Nutr.* 2017; 8(2): 213-225.

222. Shin, S., Lee, H., Kim, C., et al. Egg Consumption and Risk of Metabolic Syndrome in Korean Adults: Results from the Health Examinees Study. *Nutrients* 2017; 9(7): 6-87.

223. Bakker, E., Lee, D., Sui, X., et al. Association of Resistive Exercise, Independent of and Combined With Aerobic Exercise, With the Incidence of Metabolic Syndrome. *Mayo Clin Proc.* 2017; 92(8):1214-1222.

224. Yang, J., Christophi, C., Farioli, A., et al. Association Between Push-up Exercise Capacity and Future Cardiovascular Events Among Active Adult Men. *JAMA Netw Open.* 2019; 2(2) E188341.

225. Akhavan, T., Luhovyy, B., Brown, P., et al. Effect of premeal consumption of whey protein and its hydrolysate on food intake and postmeal glycemia and insulin response in young adults. *Am J Nutr.* 2010; 91(4): 966-975.

226. Akhavan, T., Luhovyy, B., Brown, P., et al. Effect of premeal consumption of whey protein and its hydrolysate on food intake and postmeal glycemia and insulin response in young adults. *Am J Nutr.* 2010; 91(4): 966-975.

227. Arciero, P., Bauer, D., Connelly, S., et al. Timed-daily ingestion of whey protein and exercise training reduces visceral adipose tissue mass and improves insulin resistance: the PRISE study. *J Appl. Physiol. (1985)* 2014;117(1): 1-10.

228. Sutton, E., Beyl, R., Early, K., et al. Early Time-Restricted Feeding Improves Insulin Sensitivity, Blood Pressure, and Oxidative Stress Even without Weight Loss in Men with Prediabetes. *Cell Metabolism.* 2018; 27(6): 1212-1221.

229. Gaziano, J., Hennekens, C., O'Donnell C., et al. Fasting triglycerides, high-density lipoprotein, and risk of myocardial infarction. *Circulation.* 1997; 96:2520-2525.

230. Riehle, C., Abel, E. Insulin signaling and heart failure. *Circ Res.* 2016; 118(7):1151-1169.

231. Cavalcante, P., Gregnani, M., Henrique, J., et al. Aerobic, but not Resistive Exercise Can Induce Inflammatory Pathways via Toll-Like 2 and 4: a Systematic Review. *Sports Med Open.* 2017; 3:42.

Chapter 9 References-Don't Die Young

232. King, M., Olson, S., Padbock, L., et al. Sugary food and beverage consumption and epithelial ovarian cancer risk: A population based case-control study. *BMC Cancer.* 2013; 13(1): 94.

233. Tasevska, N., Park, Y., Jiao, L., et al. Sugars and risk of mortality in the NIH-AARP Diet and Health Study. *Am J. Clin Nutr.* 2014; 99(5): 1077-1088.

234. Calle, E., Kaaks, R. Overweight, obesity, and cancer: epidemiological evidence and proposed mechanisms. *Nat Rev Cancer.* 2004; 4(8): 579-591.

235. Ausk, K., Boyko, E., Ioannou, G. Insulin resistance predicts mortality in nondiabetic individuals in the U.S. *Diabetes Care.* 2010; 33(6): 1179-1185.

236. Tsujimoto, T., Kajio, H., Sugiyama, T., et al. Association between hyperinsulinemia and increased risk of cancer death in nonobese and obese people: A population-based observational study. *Int. J Cancer.* 2017; 141(1): 102-111.

237. Trevisan, M., Liu, J., Muti, P., et al. Markers of insulin resistance and colorectal cancer mortality. *Cancer Epidemiol. Biomarkers Prev.* 2001; 10(9): 937-941.

238. Perseghin, G., Calori, G., Lattuada, G., et al. Insulin resistance/hyperinsulinemia and cancer mortality: the Cremona study at the 15th year of follow-up. *Acta Diabetol.* 2012; 49(6): 421-428.

239. Kakehi, E., Kotani, K., Nakamura, T., et al. Non-diabetic Glucose levels and Cancer Mortality: A Literature Review. *Current Diabetes Rev.* 2017; July 11.

240. Cho, D., Jang, J., Kim, S., et al. Site-specific cancer risk in people with type 2 diabetes: Nationwide population-based cohort study in Korea. *Endocrine Abstracts.* 2017; 49:EP438.

241. Ryu, T., Park, J., Scherer, P. Hyperglycemia as a Risk Factor for Cancer Progression. *Diabetes Metab J.* 2014; 38(5): 330-336.

242. Longo, V., Fontana, L. Calorie restriction and cancer prevention: metabolic and molecular mechanisms. *Trends Pharmacol Science.* 2010; 31(2): 89-98.

243. Aubrey, B., Kelly, G., Janic, A., et al. How does p53 induce apoptosis and how does this relate to p53-mediated tumor suppression? *Cell Death Differ.* 2018; 25(1):104-113.

244. Wolf, J., Lei, G., Varadhachary, A., et al. Oral lactoferrin results in T-cell dependent tumor inhibition of head and neck squamous cell carcinoma in viva. *Clin Cancer Res.* 2007; 13(5):1601-1610.

245. Slattery, M., Curtin, K., Ma, K., et al. Diet activity, and lifestyle associations with p53 mutations in colon tumors. *Cancer Epidemiol Biomarkers Prev.i* 2002; 11(6):541-548.

246. Strycharz, J., Drzewoski, J., Szemraj, J., et al. Is p53 involved in tissue specific insulin resistance formation? *Oxid Med Cell Longev.* 2017; 2017:9270549.

247. LaGory, E., Giaccia, A., A low-carb diet kills tumor cells with a mutant p53 tumor suppressor gene. *Cell Cycle.* 2013; 12(5):718-719.

248. Prokesch, A., Graef, F., Madl, T., et al. Liver p53 is stabilized upon starvation and required for amino acid catabolism and gluconeogenesis. *FASEB J.* 2017; 31(2):732-742.

249. Chen, S., Yi, Y., Hong, Z., et al. The influences of red wine in phenotype of human cancer cells. *Gene.* 2018; S0378-1119(18) 31086-2.

250. Wallenborg, K., Vlachos, P., Eriksson, S., et al. Red wine triggers cell death and thioredoxin reductase inhibition effects beyond resveratrol and SIRT1. *Exp Cell Res.* 2009; 315(8): 1360-1371.

251. Beulens, J., VanBeers, R., Stolk, R., et al. The effect of moderate alcohol consumption on fat distribution and adipocytokines. *Obesity (Silver Spring).* 2006; 14(1): 60-66.

252. Tresserra-Rimbau, A., Medina-Remón, A., Lamuela-Raventós, R., et al. Moderate red wine consumption is associated with a lower prevalence of the metabolic syndrome in the PREDIMED population. *British J Nutri.* 2015; 113(S2): S121-S130.

253. Liu, Y., Nguyen, N., Colditz, G. Links between alcohol consumption and breast cancer: a look at the evidence. *Women's Health (London).* 2015; 11(1): 65-77.

254. Gronbaek, M., Becker, U., Johansen, D., et al. Type of alcohol consumed and mortality from all causes, coronary heart disease, and cancer. *Ann Intern Med.* 2000; 133(6): 411-419.

255. Gronbaek, M., Jensen, M., Johansen, D., et al. Intake of beer, wine, and spirits, and risk of heavy drinking and alcoholic cirrhosis. *Biol Res.* 2004; 37(2): 195-200.

256. Vendelbo, M., Clasen, B., Treebak, J., et al. Insulin resistance after a 72-hour fast is associated with impaired AS-160 phosphorylation and an accumulation of lipid and glycogen in human skeletal muscle. *Am J Physiol Endocrinol Metab.* 2012; 302(2)E190-E200.

257. Schweitzer, G., Arias, E., Cartee, G. Sustained postexercise increases in AS-160 Thr642 and Ser588 phosphorylation in skeletal muscle without sustained increase in kinase phosphorylation. *J Appl Physiol (1985).* 2012; 113(12): 1852-1861.

258. Sun, M., Feng, W., Wang, F., Meta-analysis on shift work and risks of specific obesity types. *Obes Rev.* 2018; 19(1): 28-40.

259. Bescos, R., Boden, M., Jackson, A., et al. Four days of simulated shift work reduces insulin sensitivity in humans. *Acta Physiologica.* 2018; 223(2): E13039.

260. Xu, L., Zhang, J., Dai, J., et al. The Effects of Dinner-to-Bedtime and Post-Dinner Walk on Gastric Cancer Across Different Age Groups: A Multicenter Case-Control Study in Southeast China. *Medicine (Baltimore).* 2016; 95(16): E3397.

261. The friends of Mount Athos. *Times Research.* Retrieve from www.athosfriends.org.

262. Sinaki, M., Itoi, E, Wahner, H., et al. Stronger back muscles reduce the incidence of vertebral fractures: a prospective 10 year follow-up of postmenopausal women. *Bone.* 2002; 30(6): 836-841.

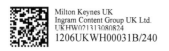